The Alkaline Diet CookBook: The Alkaline Meal Plan to Balance your pH, Reduce Body Acid, Lose Weight and Have Amazing Health

Adidas Wilson

Published by Adidas Wilson, 2017.

THE ALKALINE DIET COOKBOOK: THE ALKALINE MEAL PLAN TO BALANCE YOUR PH, REDUCE BODY ACID, LOSE WEIGHT AND HAVE AMAZING HEALTH

First edition. March 16, 2017.

Copyright © 2017 Adidas Wilson.

ISBN: 978-1393531173

Written by Adidas Wilson.

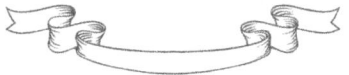

Disclaimer: The information contained in this book is intended for
educational purposes only and is not a substitute for advice, diagnosis
or treatment by a licensed physician. It is not meant to cover all
possible precautions, drug interactions, circumstances or adverse
effects. You should seek prompt medical care for any health issues and
consult your doctor before using alternative medicine or making a
change to your regimen.

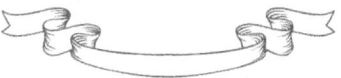

"Let food be your medicine, let medicine be your food."
- Imhotep

Table of Contents

INTRODUCTION

Introduction

A RAW FOOD DIET OCCURS when one consumes uncooked or unprocessed foods. It is also referred to as raw foodies and ensures that the consumer intakes maximum nutrients and zero additives. Raw diets are easy to digest and sort of a lifestyle which stems for raw products consumption. Simply put, it is a lifestyle that promotes real food intake in the most natural state.

Consumption of raw vegetables and fresh fruits is championed for all since it is healthy for our bodies. But there are some who fully recognize themselves as raw vegans. These are people who will consume nothing else than raw vegetables. Natural nutrients and enzymes packed in raw foods assist the body achieve optimal health levels.

Raw food normally should not have any exposure herbicides or pesticides that are genetically altered. This means that raw foods are purely organic. Raw foods should not go through any form of processing, cooking or microwaving. Such is considered unhealthy since cooking obliterates most immune boosting enzymes and vitamins in the food. Consumption of raw foods also is half the amount of calories consumed, thus a recommended diet for people looking to shed weight.

Benefits of Raw foodies

Natural enzymes in the raw diet greatly relieve of constipation, indigestion and boost the fight against chronic diseases. Raw diets boost memory and body immunity, improves diabetes and arthritis and cures headaches and allergies. Integrating raw diets in your meals will see an improved control in weight and long term exemptions of chronic illnesses.

Raw foodies help in clearing up of skin, preventing nutritional deficiencies while providing more dietary fiber. Raw diets are a good shield against cancer, assists in keeping the liver functioning optimally and maintain a healthy heart. A diet of raw foods lowers inflammation, gives the body more energy and reduces the risk of consuming carcinogens and anti-nutrients.

Raw foods also come in handy in reducing and preventing acidity while building on the alkaline blood pH balance. These kinds of raw foods are recommended for people struggling with high cholesterol and high blood pressure. The raw food diet is also recommendable to curing hormonal imbalances, kidney diseases, and bladder or gallstone complications. Fatigue, muscle aches and painful joints are also catered for by consuming raw foods.

The intake of raw food assists in the much required body cleansing. This is because raw foods take a shorter time to digest. The shorter time taken to digest food improves the body's ability to exempt toxemia and fermentation of waste in the colons.

Risks of Raw Food Diets on your Health

A good number of people on raw diets will repulse to eating animal products, which are sources of vitamins. If they do not eat other vitamin supplements, it is likely they would suffer from vitamin deficiencies. There is also the risk of over reliance on certain types of foods which will mostly lead to the denial of particular nutrients and enzymes in the body.

How to Do it correctly

Many people relying on raw fruits and vegetables only end up having eroded teeth. Teeth erode as a result of acids from fruits and vegetables eating up the teeth enamel. The sugars of the fruit and the gum of dried fruit stick to the teeth causing rot.

Quality minerals, antioxidants and vitamins come from fresh organic fruits and vegetables, especially when consumed. However there is a significant need for balancing the intake of raw foods with meat, fish and steamed foods so as to remain healthy.

1.

What is Alkaline Diet and why it Matters

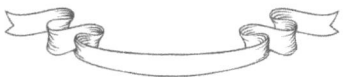

A HUMAN BODY IS PRONE to all sorts of problems, and most of them anchored on diet issues. One of these problems is the acidosis, which results from the lack of balanced PH level. It is in this situation where an alkaline diet comes in, to help you develop a better balance of these levels, besides helping in many other factors that are central to your health. So, is an alkaline diet that important really and how does it help? Here are several things you should know about alkaline diet and how it helps in providing an optimal balance of such crucial aspect of the human existence.

Effects of lack of alkaline diet

One of the major results of lack of an alkaline diet is the imbalance in PH, leading to more acid in the blood. This prevents absorption minerals and other nutrients, besides deterring the body's ability to heal itself. The body PH is central to almost everything. The lack of this determinant and the consecutive acidosis leads to several health complications as immunity deficiencies, digestive problems, heart conditions and kidney diseases as well as accelerated aging, to mention just a few.

How can an alkaline diet help?

One and significant effect of alkaline diet is to provide the PH balance needed, which helps cut the cycle of retrieving the balance from the cells, which leads to them becoming acidic and developing diseases. Besides, with an ample balance, diseases caused by bacteria and cancerous cells cannot get the opportunity to take root in your body if you have been observing proper alkaline diet. This is because these causative agents thrive in acidic body conditions. With sufficient supply of alkaline foods, the body can be able to heal itself from toxins and heavy metals among other predicaments that come with the absence of this inevitable diet.

● **Benefits of alkaline diet**

Several benefits accrue to supply of alkaline-rich minerals. This includes, among others, protection of the bone density and muscle mass, based on the development of bone structure and sustaining muscles as aging checks in. The other significant benefit is a small risk of hypertension and stroke, resulting from sustainable cardiovascular health and low cholesterol, all thanks to the availability of alkaline in the body. Additionally, you can also count on alkaline sufficiency if you are seeking to reduce cases of chronic pain in the back, headache and joint pain among others, which result from chronic acidosis.

As there is plenty of alkalizing vegetables and fruits, you can always try to fight this problem without necessarily having to go through complicated medical procedures. You can get these veggies or fruits from the store and get the adequate intake required to keep you healthy and safe. This is one of the dietary necessities usually taken for granted, but as much as you keep working on other diet-controlled factors, you need to remember that the results of lack of a sustaining flow of alkalizing diet can cost you a big deal, even your life. If you have not yet considered this diet, then the time is now, you have to do something before it is too late.

2.

Reducing acidity in your body

ACIDIC AND ALKALINE levels are indicated in your body through pH scales. Alkaline levels in your blood should be maintained ideally at or between the pH ranges of 7.35 – 7.45. At the ranges of 7.35, your body is highly acidic and prone to a variety of illnesses. Consumption of highly acidic foods strains minerals such as Calcium, Magnesium, Potassium and Sodium from the bone deposits by regulating the acid levels.

Acidosis has some universal symptoms such as difficulty in breathing (or running out of breath), cold feet or hands, heartburn, reduced sex drive, a metallic taste in your mouth, mucus build up, chemical sensitivity, joint and muscular pains. Any of the above symptoms could be pointing out probabilities of body acidity.

What to do to Decrease Body Acidity

There are a number of do's and don'ts to cater to body acidity. Continuous consumption of foods that promote alkalinity in your body is a plus. Foods that are classified as alkaline include broccoli, celery, avocados, pepper and kale. The products mentioned assist in maintaining and sustaining a pH balanced diet. Alkalized diets are mostly consisted of fruits and vegetables which create bicarbonates that wade off acidosis. The foods also help in maintaining and sustaining bone strength in the body, as opposed to the foods containing animal products and grains.

Avoiding processed and canned foods also promotes alkaline levels in the body. Organic products also have minimal levels of acidity. Processed foods such as dairy products, caffeine, sodas, meats, fat, alcohol, refined flours and sugars are risky foods in terms of acidity and should be avoided at all costs.

People struggling with acidity should also consider reducing their stress levels. Stress and body acid production are related. Taking deep breaths is an effective way of reducing stress levels and tension in the body. Deep breaths increase oxygen levels in the body while doing away carbon dioxide through exhalation.

Intake of alkaline water is also recommended as an effective way of cutting acidity in the blood. Alkaline water contains minerals such as potassium and calcium which are vital in reducing acidity in the body. Alkaline water is also recommended to women going through menopause because it reduces the risks of bone loss.

You can also make a homemade antacid by using baking powder (sodium bicarbonate) which contains buffering properties that counter acidity. Such neutralization of acidic levels assists in balancing acid-alkali balance. If you however have pre-existing medical issues, do consult your medical practitioner before inducing this homemade remedy.

HOME REMEDY FOR ACIDITY

Ingredients

- 1/3 teaspoon sodium bicarbonate (baking soda)
- 2 tablespoons of organic apple cider vinegar or fresh lemon squeeze

Directions

Mix all the ingredients together. The mixture will start fizzing.

When the fizzing subsides, add 8 ounces of water.

Drink the mixture in a single gulp.

The remedy is able to restore blood and body pH balance levels. It also helps in the reduction of stomach acidity and acidosis.

For optimal actualization of the acid-alkali balance and balanced levels of pH balance, it is advisable to intertwine the alkaline diets with body exercises.

3.

WATERMELON CLEANSE

FRUIT CLEANSING IS a great way to get rid of the extra toxins gained after a brief period of unhealthy eating. By detoxifying your body of the harmful toxins you can start a healthy lifestyle and follow a diet plan to suit your daily needs.

Due to unhealthy eating habits, over a period of time, the body tends to accumulate a lot of toxins. These toxins are harmful to the health and may affect the individual at a later stage in life. Youngsters may gobble up on any food they find and not get sick by that as their metabolism demands a continuous food supply. But as the body ages, even people from 30 years of age start to feel the necessity to get rid of the toxins they have accumulated over the years.

The process of getting rid of these toxins is called as Body Cleansing or Detox.

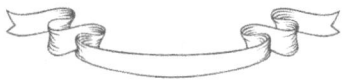

WATERMELON CLEANSING:

Watermelon cleansing is one such form of a detoxifying agent which can help is systematically removing the toxins from various organs like the liver, kidney, colon, etc.

Let us see what are the different ways we can carry out watermelon cleanse:

1. Eating:

This is the best way to start. Just bring a big watermelon and gorge on it. The best part about watermelon is that it has 90% water in it. You can just eat it without feeling hungry or thirsty. Watermelon is very juicy and is simply very refreshing. One big watermelon may be sufficient for most but if your appetite is big, you can always eat a bit more.

This cleansing technique depends on the amount of detox you plan. Normally, this diet is recommended for 1 or 2 days. Not more than that. It is recommended that you eat watermelon at regular intervals instead of eating your tummy full in a single time. Schedule your day as per 4 meals.

Note: Try not to put the watermelon in the fridge. It is better if eaten at room temperature.

1. Juice:

Another simple method of the diet is by making a juice and drinking it after regular intervals. Many people tend to discard the rind of the watermelon and then eat the fruit. But the rind is very important for the body. The rind contains higher quantities of minerals and amino acids. It can also help in balancing the sweetness of the watermelon.

When you make watermelon juice, the rind can be crushed in the fruit and the minerals and amino acids will not be lost. This is the main advantage of the juice diet.

It is recommended that for such a diet and Organic Watermelon is preferred.

Also, the juice too should be taken at regular intervals in appropriate quantities. You can divide the day into in meals.

3. Smoothies:

You can also mix chopped pieces of watermelon with the juice. Drinking only juice or eating only the fruit can be a bit monotonous, so a smoothie is a perfect blend for a diet. You can even add the seeds as the seeds contain fiber and also zinc. Add one or two cubes of ice to make it more refreshing.

Smoothies too are to be had at regular intervals throughout the day.

1. Hybrid:

If you think that eating watermelon or drinking its juice is a bit boring then you can experiment with different hybrid recipes involving other fruits but it must be remembered that watermelon must always be the hero of the recipe.

This may lessen the intensity of the detoxification but still you will get good results if you are adding appropriate ingredients.

Mix healthy substitutes and you will be just fine.

WHY WATERMELON?

All fruits are healthy and are great to carry out a cleansing diet with them but watermelon is extra special. First of all, it has high water content. Every detox diet will ask you to drink 2-3 liters of water and what better than to drink the same in the form of a fruit. More you drink water more frequently will you take a pee. This is very useful in detox.

One of the primary health benefits of watermelon is to improve the kidney function. It is also known to treat kidney stones and infections of the urinary tract. Another great advantage is specifically for the male readers. Watermelon contains citrulline, which is the main ingredient of the drug Viagra.

Watermelon has the highest concentration of an important antioxidant, Lycopene, than any other fruit.

Due to all these benefits, watermelon is one of the best fruit for body cleansing.

If carried out successfully it is the best form of cleansing to get your body detoxified after some holidays and get back to following a healthy lifestyle.

NOTE:

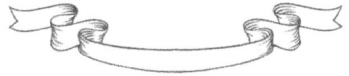

WATERMELON DIET IS recommended only for 1 or 2 days. Also, in some of the cases, it is not even recommended. This depends on person to person and such a diet should only be carried out under the advice of the doctor.

4.

All you need for an Alkalizing Diet

WITH THE BODY'S PH level maintenance being an inevitable survival necessity, going for an alkalizing diet is almost the only natural option for humankind. Although the kidneys are working so hard to ensure that this balance is maintained, a proper diet is necessary to make sure that everything is put under control, since a slight failure may lead to kidney problems.

There is a broad range of foods that can be used to provide this critical input. Therefore, only people's ignorance can lead them to problems. Here are several foods you can include in your plan to ensure sufficient alkalizing diet for your body.

1. Go green

If you are looking for an alkalizing diet option, then vegetables are for you. All vegetables are good in this field. Therefore, all you need is to take lots and lots of them. However, for the veggies to be helpful, they should be eaten as natural as possible, either raw or steamed. Some of these vegetables include kale, spinach, parsley, seaweed and watercress among others.

1. Eat enough fruits

Fruits are also important for alkalizing, leave for a few such as plums, blueberries, and cranberries, which are known to be acidifying. Just like the vegetables, taking fruits raw can help in getting the best of their nutritional content. Besides, they should be natural rather than processed. Something fascinating about some fruits is that Apple cider vinegar is alkalizing, despite Vinegar being famous for its acidity.

1. Have you tried the legumes yet?

Although not all grains are alkalizing, such types as millet, quinoa, fresh beans, green peas, green soy, and amaranth are an excellent source of this essential nutrient. However, as it is the case with nuts and seeds, you can always soak and sprout whole grains and the beans to make them alkalizing.

1. Foods that you need to avoid

Although it is a regular phenomenon to have some alkalizing and acidifying foods, there are foods you need to steer well clear if you are looking for the alkalizing type. One of these food types is animal produce, especially meat. Others include poultry and dairy products, as well as fish, although fish are quite better off than the others are. Moreover, if you have been keeping processed foods at bay, you are on the right track. One of the notorious agents of acidifying foods are artificial sweeteners, which are prevalent in processed foods, one good example is the white sugar.

Primarily, the feature of either acidifying or alkalizing in food depends on the amount of acid that is produced as a by-product of its digestion. The acidic waste is what has an effect on the body, and not the acidity of the food itself. However, with this in mind, it is also very useful to make use of our knowledge on which food are acidifying and the ones on the alkalizing side in making diet decisions. If you know the importance of an alkalizing diet or the effects of lack of enough alkalizing components in the body, then you would not hesitate to go for what is best for you.

5.

Signs of too much acid in your body

ACIDOSIS HAS A VARIETY of telltale signs that one can easily pin point out in their everyday life. First and foremost is when you are on a diet yet nagging cravings for a particular food, waking up tired after having a superb night is also a potential risk of too much acid in your blood pH balance.

Unhealthy eating will at most instance leave you feeling fatigued, sluggish and heavily lazy all over. Evidence has proven that people who are overweight, fatigued, stressed, have reflux, bad skin, struggling with indigestion, and complain of muscle and joint pains suffer from acidosis. Detailed scrutiny of people with above mentioned complications always had one common cue, acid imbalance in their blood pH levels.

Acid is corrosive and can burn through metals. With that in mind it is horrific to think what it could be doing to your body from the inside. If acidosis remains unchecked it will definitely eat you up alive. Acid will surely corrode your cardiovascular system, erode your joints and kill your digestive system. Thus anyone going through such bodily complications should immediately start an alkaline diet to balance their pH blood balance.

Stop Suicidal Eating Habits

Daily consumption of processed sugars and flour, gluten, meats, caffeine, carbonated water or sodas, artificial sweeteners, and processed foods is not healthy for you. Awkwardly, these foods are the most sought after in the world today. More and more people are hooked on acidosis due to unhealthy eating habits, even in the developing and third world countries.

Toxic elements and acid accumulate in one's body rapidly, these coupled with stress builds massive inflammation in the body and joints. This inflammation drains out the body's energy since the body has to fight hard to stay afloat. That in itself is the sole reason why you wake every morning too fatigued for comfort.

Most people want to quickly mend their fatigue with caffeine and thus take large quantities of energy boosts, sugars, coffee among others. This in turn heightens their reliance on the acidic stimulants and in the end they cannot sleep. They are simply too uncomfortable in their own bodies.

It is however possible to turn all this around, but it won't be an overnight event. It takes both will and hard work to reverse the effects of acidosis in the blood pH balance. It is a worthy investment, consisting of adding up small things in your diet that change everything. It does not translate to your depriving or cutting off everything that you enjoy.

Breathing is common to all people, but many are faced with respiratory ease due to acidosis. To counter the effects of acidosis, it is recommended that you have breathing exercises three times per day. Inhaling oxygen refreshes all your body organs. When exhaling, carbon dioxide is let out. Carbon dioxide is over a hundred times more acidic than any other component in the body. Releasing carbon dioxide is thus a plus for a healthier you.

Drinking or eating more fresh vegetables and fruits is another effective way to combating acidosis. This is because the vegetables and fruits are entirely alkaline in nature, therefore assisting in balancing the blood pH balance.

6.

How to Make a Creamy Avocado Gazpacho

AVOCADO IS A HEALTHY and tasty fruit that can be used in various ways, and can as well be used with veggies and other fruits, thanks to its versatility. However, there is always something special about taking avocado separately, especially if you decide to make a creamy gazpacho, you can never go wrong with this fruit.

Benefits of Avocado

One good thing about the avocado is that it is high in Omega-9 fatty acid, which is in the form of monounsaturated fat. Also known as, the oleic acid, this fat is not considered an essential fatty acid like others due to the inability of our bodies to make it in large amounts. It is, therefore, important that you supplement this essential yet rare component by including avocado and other foods high in it in your diet.

Besides, avocados are also vital for the heart, brain, skin, hair, and slowing down signs of aging among other benefits. They are also rich in fiber, which is readily soluble and helps in lowering cholesterol and maintaining blood sugar. Avocados are packed with vitamin E, which is helpful in regulating inflammation. This fruit is also rich in essential alkaline minerals like Magnesium and Potassium.

Here is a simple step-by-step recipe on making Avocado Gazpacho that you may find useful if you need to make something flavorful, quick and healthy without having to cook.

Avocado Gazpacho

Yield

Serves 2
Ingredients
2 Haas avocados
1 small zucchini, chopped
2 stalks celery, chopped
½ cup cilantro
¼ cup parsley that is finely chopped
¼ cup Spanish onion, chopped
1 garlic clove, ensure it is minced
1 ½ cups of filtered water
½ jalapeno, they should be seeded and chopped
1 lime, Juiced
Some Salt and pepper
To finish, Garnish with some basil leaves and cucumber slices'
Directions
Use a processor to blend all of the ingredients; you can leave it a bit chunky or completely mushy, as you desire.

Add the salt and pepper; adjust to your preferred taste
Enjoy your creamy avocado gazpacho
Making this meal is quite simple; you can make it on-the-go, even when you do not have sufficient time to hit the kitchen for some tedious cooking process. Even better, it features significant advantages that you may not find with most cooked foods or processed ones. If you do not have sufficient time to make something from the kitchen, this could be a better option that you can prepare faster than processed foods that will doom your health.

The avocado is also classified as alkaline foods, so if you have been taking acidic foods of late, you may give yourself a break by grabbing the avocado gazpacho to balance your PH level. The other advantages will follow, all you need to do is try it out and find out what the avocado is capable of doing for your health.

7.

YOUR IDEAL WHOLE FOODS Diet Plan to Lose Weight

When it comes to weight loss, how you work your way there are sometimes all that matters. You may have all the options with you, but having a great diet plan counts in achieving the results you are craving. In that case, nothing works any better than a good whole food diet plan, especially when you are into losing weight. This plan has to do with scheduling your meals appropriately, which helps avoid taking too many additional meals, rather, you can be able to take only a few fulfilling meals in a day. Here are several ways in which you can plan your diet and make it quite easy.

What is best for breakfast?

Taking a whole food satisfying breakfast keeps you off the dishes for the better part of the day. This meal should not comprise of processed foods with additives and sweeteners. For instance, taking Greek yogurt, which has plenty of protein, can help you get over the urges to take any bites in the morning hours. Only go for a plain and non-fat variety, and then you can sweeten it by adding some fruits. Alternatively, you can go for steel-cut oats, which have more fiber but avoid the flavored types that may contain sugars. A cup of green tea can be good too.

During lunch or dinner

This is the ideal time to take a nourishing meal. Go for foods from whole grains, and some healthy proteins as poultry and fish. You should also ensure to bring on board some vegetables like Broccoli, Spinach. You can also take some lean ham, low-fat bacon, reduced-fat sausages, and nuts as part of the mains dish. All these can help keep you sufficiently fueled throughout the day, or keep you off the cabinets later at night.

When preparing some desserts

Having to take whole foods to lose weight does not rule out the possibility of getting treats with desserts whatsoever. Besides, there are still healthy desserts that you can still enjoy and keep your weight under check. A fruit salad with some berries or fresh coconut can be a great treat. If you like butternut, you can have some of its squash, mixed with an avocado or cinnamon, and topped with some cocoa powder or honey, or both for a healthy taste.

When you need some snack

Whole food snacks are good for you, not only for the nutrition that you need but also for sustaining you and reducing overeating when you get to your main meals. Many snacks around can give you the quality you need without necessarily compromising your efforts to lose weight. Some snacks as unsweetened raisins, banana chips, dehydrated green beans and dried apple rings can be perfect for between the meals bites if you feel that you have to take some.

Planning wisely can help you maneuver through the maze of weight loss tactics and make it easy. If you can keep these tips within your reach, it is evident that you will find it fascinating how you can lose weight effortlessly by just eating healthy. That is how the use of whole foods in achieving weight loss plays the trick; you can try it out and see for yourself.

8.

WHY WHOLE FOODS ARE your Best Weight Loss Option

Weight loss comes with its costs, whether you have to cut on a diet or go the hard way and hit the exercise route. However, this does not have to be the case; you do not have to starve yourself or workout all day to reduce your waistline, not with whole foods option at your disposal. Many varieties of these foods are out there and can help you reduce fat so effortlessly and seamlessly. There are several reasons why whole foods stand out as the best choice for people who are struggling with the weight predicament and here are some of them.

Why whole foods and how do they work?

SEVERAL REASONS MAKE whole foods qualify as the ideal choice for weight loss. First, these foods help burn excessive fat, which is a major contributor to weight gain. By enhancing your body's metabolism, fat stored in body's reservoirs as the tummy and in the waistline is burnt and reduced. What's more, taking whole meals lead to feeling fed without going beyond the calorie intake line. This is a great way of ensuring that you prevent weight gain, as you fight with losing the current extra weight. Additionally, taking a good meal with sufficient level of whole foods helps keep your urge for food in check, which means you do not have to hit the shelves for snacks (which may be one of the leading causes of weight gain) now and then.

What are some of the best Whole Foods?

With the wide variety of these foods at your disposal, only you can be so reluctant as not to make use of their availability and change the course of fighting the excess weight. Look at such foods that help burn fat as whole grain oats, beans, lentils, almonds (milk, butter), eggs, spinach, and Broccoli, to mention just a few. All these foods can be far reaching in effect if you are into burning fat with your diet. More importantly, when dealing with grains, go for the whole grain foods, since they are better than the ground and processed ones.

What Foods Should I Avoid?

Well, as much as many whole foods may be significant in weight loss, some of them may not be as friendly if they are processed. In cases of grains, you need to keep your intake of processed foods at bay. Although made from whole food ingredients, the manufacturers may add additives and sweeteners that can drastically thwart your goals in achieving weight loss with whole foods. It is, therefore, imperative to stay well clear of artificial foods, whether or not they are processed from whole foods.

At the bottom line, we can agree that achieving weight loss with whole foods is easier than you may think. However, it is not that this way of losing weight does not come with its sacrifices, where you may have to cut back on that favorite snack, cheese or chocolate. Although this does not mean having to do away with them completely, going slow on the artificial foods is all you can do to give enough room for the whole foods and I can assure you, the latter works wonders.

9.

Why Bulletproof Tea is all you Need

GOOD TEA IN THE MORNING may be all you need to get your day started on a high note. Whether you like coffee or another type of tea, it is always wise to ensure you take tea that can give you the necessary health requirement for your day. This is where bulletproof tea comes in; to give you not only the energy that will help you through morning hours, but also provides sufficient health benefits that you cannot overlook. Here is how you can make this simple but effective drink.

Ingredients

1 to 2 cups brewed tea (Matcha, Rooibos or Oolong)

Several tablespoons of your preferred milk (coconut, almond, goat or cow, but not soy)

1 tablespoon MCT oil

1 tablespoon butter, pastured

Directions

Brew the tea according to your preference

Add your butter in the hot teacup and cover to melt it

After completely melting, add the milk and MTC oil

Blend it to emulsify the liquid fat into the tea and milk

Enjoy your powerful drink

It is important mentioning that this drink can cause loose bowels, digestive complications, and nausea if not used correctly. Therefore, introduce it slowly over time to give your body time to adjust.

Similarly, you may like to try another type of tea, which is also bulletproof and comes with many benefits besides keeping you full through the morning. This one is ideal if you are getting up early for work, or a morning workout.

Ingredients

1 inch of fresh turmeric, sliced

1 inch fresh ginger, sliced

1 tbsp. coconut oil

500 ml coconut or almond milk

1 tsp cinnamon, powdered

1 tsp maca, powdered

1 tsp coconut or rice malt syrup

Directions

Slice your turmeric and ginger, and then put them in a saucepan together with your milk, cinnamon, coconut oil, maca and the syrup (optional).

Let simmer and leave it to cook for about 5 more minutes, or 10 minutes if you like, to give the ginger and turmeric more time to spread.

Blend them in a high power appliance for about 30 sec on high speed to ensure the ginger and turmeric liquefy to achieve a smooth froth.

Serve Your Tea and Enjoy

One thing about this tea is that it will give you the kick to keep going for hours. It can sustain you for up to four or five hours before you think of grabbing a plate or snack. What's more important, if you are doing something that necessitates concentration like writing or such, this drink is for you. It will keep your mind focused and clear, which is an essential tone for starting your day. This means you can stay focused throughout the day.

If you have not tried this tea yet, then the time is now; you need to check it out and see its benefits for yourself, you will love it. Besides, it is also a great drink to prepare for your family in the morning as well, but keep in mind that for the first option, you should maintain the advance of the fat steady to get your body used to the changes.

10.

Five Benefits of Sage you need to see for yourself

ONE OF THE MOST OUTSTANDING features of Sage is that it is capable of treating most ailments. From simple skin conditions, digestion regulations to the complicated problems like chronic diseases and cognitive disorders. Sage has leaves that are used for medicinal purposes, and it comes with many benefits, more than it is credited for in most cases. Here are some of its advantages.

1. Cognitive Benefits

Sage has proved to be an excellent solution for memory retention. The herb is also vital for brain activity with an increase in concentration and focus. This is far reaching in brain boosting, which is crucial for the young and the aging alike. It can be taken by sniffing or consumption by adding it to your diet.

2. Immune Boosting

Sage contains antimicrobial qualities in sage that are very helpful in prevention of bacterial and viral infections that can find their way into the body through the skin. The herb can be applied by the use of a cream or antibacterial use for protection against such illness factors.

3. Inflammation

Although the flavor from sage make it difficult to chew its leaves, this method may be essential to get the herb working faster than with other forms. Sage is efficient in fighting inflammation in respiratory and gastrointestinal tracts, as well as a remedy for other problems like arthritis, gout and the cardiovascular system inflammation, which can result in heart diseases or blood pressure. This is all thanks to sage components like phenolic and flavonoids.

4. Antioxidants

Problems from free radicals resulting from hazard by-products of metabolism in cells attacking healthy cells can spell doom for your health. These include chronic conditions and degenerative diseases that you need to keep away for as long as you can. The good news is that sage has antioxidant properties like luteolin, rosmarinic and apigenin that can neutralize these radicals to prevent creation of oxidative stress in critical organs like the heart, joints, skin, brain and the heart among others.

5. Boosting Bone Strength

Sage has one component that is never taken serious, vitamin k; this vitamin is very useful in the body, and is not popular in many foods. It is essential for bone density development and bone integrity as aging sets in. If you have not been working on ensuring better bone health, or have been on sedentary lifestyle with poor nutrient intake, then you should consider increasing your sage intake to boost your vitamin k levels. You can add sage leaves in your diet, which will give you about 27% of the required daily intake.

Sage may not be taken as a useful herb, but it has more to offer than it is considered. It is, therefore, time you considered going for this useful way of treating notorious problems. It may not be as demanding or expensive as the medicines you would otherwise seek, but it will give you more than you need to get many of the health problems sorted.

11.

Benefits of Cayenne Pepper

CAYENNE PEPPER HAS been in use in many societies from the beginning of time. It has been used therapeutically, but cayenne also stands as a reliable component for cleansing and detoxifying among other purposes. Here are several benefits of cayenne pepper.

Migraine Headache

Cayenne has been helpful in preventing migraine headache. This is due to its ability to trigger a pain response in another part of the body, which redirects the brain's attention to the new area. This condition leads to nerve fibers depleting substance P, resulting in reduced pain.

Supporting Digestion

This pepper is not only useful for seasoning food but also helps in digestion by stimulating tee digestive tract, which leads to increased enzyme and gastric juices production. This, in turn, facilitates the ability of the body to metabolize foods and toxins easier and faster. Cayenne also helps in reducing the effects of intestinal gas by stimulating intestinal movement for better assimilation and elimination.

Anticancer Agent

According to a study in Loma Linda in California, this pepper is capable of preventing lung cancer among smokers. This is thanks to cayenne's compound known as capsaicin, which is a substance that is capable of preventing the growth of tobacco-induced tumors. In other studies, this pepper has proved to have similar resistance against liver tumors.

Weight Loss Aid

Research has shown that when taken for breakfast, cayenne helps prevent appetite, which leads to reduced calorie intake. Besides, with its metabolism support, this pepper helps in burning excess fats in the body.

Blood Clot Prevention

By reducing atherosclerosis, cayenne aids in fibrinolytic activity, thus preventing factors that can contribute in blood clots forming in the body. This reduction in blood clot helps in reducing the risk of heart attack or stroke.

Detoxing

As a renowned circulatory stimulant, you can expect cayenne to have something positive about the lymphatic system. Well, this spice does not only help with this function but also helps increase lymphatic pulse and the rhythm of digestion. This leads to heating of the body, which is useful for the detoxification process. Besides, through promoting sweating, cayenne helps in detoxification further through the process. For total body detox, mix it with lemon juice and honey, and you got good tea for the purpose.

Heart Health

By keeping blood pressure at normal levels, and balancing the body's level of LDL cholesterol, cayenne helps achieve a healthy heart condition. This pepper also assists in the optimization of triglycerides, which is also vital in ensuring a healthy heart.

It is not just about the taste, or the way cayenne makes your food taste; there is more to this pepper than you would expect. If you are having any of these problems, but you do not know where to start, you may be spared the struggle of going to the doctor since you have the remedy that can come in handy at your disposal. However, you can use this pepper for keeping healthy, but it does not mean you should not seek medical attention in case of a serious problem. Go ahead and enjoy your cayenne pepper, and take advantage of its useful effects on various parts of your body.

12.

Benefits of Cloves You Probably did Not Know

LIKE MOST SPICES, CLOVES have their fair share of popularity in the kitchen, but it also has some spectacular qualities that make it a necessity in the medicinal industry. Cloves come from flower buds of trees from Indonesia's native rainforest. Cloves have this tasty and flavor rich quality but are high in components that can be useful for medication as well.

How to Select and Store

Cloves are available in groceries throughout the year. If they are of high quality, these buds should have this fragrant smell upon squeezing. Go for the buds rather than clove powder, since the latter may not be pure. In selecting the buds, it is also wise to ensure they have the stem and sepals intact, and they are whole. You can store your cloves in a closed container and keep them in cool dark place. This way they can last for longer. You can also grind cloves with a hand mill. If you have clove powder, store it in a refrigerator, inside containers that are airtight. However, clove powder should not be kept for long, as it is vulnerable to losing its flavor over a short time than the bud type.

Benefits of Cloves

1. Remedy for Respiratory Infections

Cloves help in reducing or preventing colds and flu. This spice can also suffice as an expectorant, which makes it ease a cough by helping release phlegm. Besides, in its natural form, the clove can act as a painkiller, as well as helping attack germs, which also assist in the fight against a sore throat.

2. Reducing Inflammation

When used for massaging sore muscles, it can bear significant relief. It is also utilized in some cases for treating rheumatism and arthritis.

3. Improving Digestion

With its ability to ease tension in the lining of the GI tract, clove helps counter vomiting, intestinal gas, diarrhea, and stomachache. However, moderation should be observed, as the spice is robust enough to cause stomach irritation.

4. Treat Bruises

Cloves are also very handy when it comes to treating scrapes and bruises. However, it can cause sting sensation, so you may need to use it along with some olive oil.

5. Relief from Toothache

If you have ever experienced pain on your tooth, then you know how far it can go when it starts taking a toll on you. However, this does not have to be excruciating if you have clove oil. If you are having extreme tooth pain, you can put clove oil on it or the gum around it with cotton and the pain will decline. Even better, if you have a problem of infection, then clove will also reduce that as well.

The next time you step into a grocery store, you have a reason to remember picking clove as you pick other essentials. Remember, excessive consumption of clove can result in central nervous system disorder, or gastrointestinal irritation. Additional problems can also cause ulcers, ulcerative colitis or diverticulitis.

13.

Blueberry Alkaline Blast for the Mornings

THIS ALKALINE SMOOTHIE is packed with, antioxidants, 4 complete sources, 6 benefiting fats, numerous vitamins and immeasurable minerals. It is a delicious power pack, healthy and immune booster that is recommended for every morning to all. The puree is a perfect fit for people dealing with yeast imbalance. There should at least be two or three healing fat sources as to effectively battle the Candida, coupled with zero or low sugar fruit.

It is also recommendable for those who are hit by hunger pains almost as immediately as they have their breakfast. This smoothie will assist anyone because the puree has certain fats which give a fulfilling effect.

Blueberry Morning Blast

Serves one

Ingredients

½ cup of blueberries

1 tablespoon chia

1 tablespoon flaxseed, ground

1 tablespoon raw almond butter

1 tablespoon coconut oil

1 tablespoon ground hemp plant seed

1 cup of coconut milk

A sizeable handful of spinach

Directions

Put the ingredients together in your choice of blending appliance.

Puree to your desired consistency.

Enjoy the delicious healthy blend.

Nutrients and Minerals in the above Alkali Puree

Spinach is low in fats at an exceptional 14%, closely followed by proteins at 30%. The rest 56% is pure carbohydrates. The low protein margins are an assurance for the alkaline nature of the vegetable. Spinach is very low in cholesterol and saturated fats; it also is a great source of zinc and niacin. Spinach is a reliable source for dietary fiber, protein, magnesium and phosphorus. There also notable deposits of calcium, copper and manganese minerals in spinach. Vitamins A, C, D and K are also present in the spinach vegetable. The vegetable is thus vital for an alkaline puree in the morning.

Hemp seed is high in dietary fiber, rich in trace minerals and vital amino acids. The seeds are particularly nutritious and rich in protein, healthy fats and a variety of minerals. The seeds are technically considered as nuts and carry a mild, nut flavor. The hemp seeds are often referred as hemp hearts. Hemp seeds are a source of vitamin E and minerals such as sulphur, zinc, sodium, magnesium, phosphorus, calcium, iron and potassium.

The Nuts in the Alkaline Morning Blast

Hemp seeds contain nitric oxide, a gas molecule which dilates and relaxes blood vessels, channeling to low blood pressure and limited risk of heart diseases. Hemp seed aide in decreasing the risk of formation blood clot and assists the heart rapid recovery in case of a heart attack. Hemp seeds contain high levels of GLA, and studies have exhibited that hemp seeds help in the reduction in the symptoms of menopause among women.

Coconuts are very nutritious and rich in fiber. The fruit also carries vitamins C, E, B1, B3, B5 and B6 coupled with minerals including iron, magnesium, phosphorous, calcium, selenium and sodium. Contrary to ordinary milk, coconut milk is lactose free so it is utilized as a milk substitute especially by people who are lactose intolerant. Fresh coconut spoils in short durations and must be consumed immediately used after pressing.

14.

Health benefits of Rosemary, Why You Should Try It

AMONG OTHER HERBS, the rosemary has its advantages that any medical practitioner would recommend for you. The herb goes a long way into helping people with various health complications. You can also grow this useful plant at home and take advantage of its strong components whenever you need it. Here are several ways on how to handle it, as well as benefits of the rosemary.

How to grow Rosemary

You can start by planting either the seeds or small rosemary plant in a local greenhouse, if you can use a natural one, then the better.

Ensure it is planted in a place with sufficient sunlight as the plant does well in the sun.

Water the plant occasionally to avoid overwatering it, as it doesn't require much water.

If your location has cold winter and autumn, then grow it outside in spring and summer.

How to Prepare

When harvesting, ensure you cut the spring at about 3 to 6 inches down, since cutting the tips alone won't do your plant much good.

In case you want to dry your sprigs, then tie them upside down and hang until they are ready or use a food dehydrator. The best part is that this plant dries quite faster, and does not lose its potency during the process.

Benefits

1. Immunity Boosting

Rosemary is high in anti-inflammatory, antioxidants and anticarcinogenic components. These features enable the plant to fight different diseases and pathogens that are a hazard to the immune system and the body in general. Antioxidants are in a secondary form of the body's defense, and these are significant in rosemary plant, with such compounds as caffeic acid, carnosol, rosmarinic acid and betulinic acid.

2. Remedy for Stomach Upsets

This plant has been used in many cultures as a remedy for upset stomach, diarrhea, bloating and constipation among other digestive problems. This is all thanks to its anti-inflammatory components and stimulant effects, which qualifies it as a solution for regulating bowel movements and gastrointestinal system.

3. Blood Flow Stimulation

Among the many advantages of rosemary in the body are its paramount benefits like boosting the production of red blood cells production, body stimulation and helping in blood flow. This is vital in helping oxygenation of vital organs and body systems as well as boosting metabolic activities in such areas. Besides, it also supports the movement of nutrients to worn out cells for repair.

4. Memory Boosting

Rosemary has long helped as a cognitive stimulant. It is necessary for increased focus and intelligence, and its effect on memory retention has been outstanding. The plant has also proved useful in stimulating cognitive activity in the elderly and people suffering from acute cognitive disorders like dementia and Alzheimer's.

5. Antibacterial

Rosemary is not only effective in boosting the immune system, but also comes in handy when it comes to fighting against bacterial infections, especially in the stomach. This plant has proved effective against H, pylori bacteria, which is a dangerous pathogen for causing stomach ulcers. It has also shown to be effective against Staph infection, which is responsible for thousands of deaths yearly.

Making a simple rosemary tea may make the difference for you. If you considered this plant just another herb, well, now you have a reason to try it and take advantage of its benefits.

15.

The Benefits of a Healthy Green Zinger Alkaline Juice

WITH MANY PEOPLE DRINKING acidic juice, it is undeniable that they are giving their stomachs a difficult task to break food down into the hydrochloric acid. This process could instead have been done simply with sodium bicarbonate. This digestive difficulty, among other problems resulting from too much consumption of acidic foods, is what makes it necessary to consider going for an alkaline drink for a healthier digestion.

Bringing Your Body Back to Alkaline State

Your body's PH is the measure of its alkaline or acidic state. This level has to be maintained at an optimum level, which calls for hard work in the body to reduce the effects of the acidic food that people eat almost every day. This is where green zinger alkaline juice comes in, to assist in restoring the desired level of your body PH.

Besides the chemical effect, green juices are also known to go a long way in cleansing your liver, blood, digestive tract and kidneys as well as supporting the major body organs. Green juices are also low in sugar as compared to fruit juice, which spares you the risk of high glycemic index that can take a toll on your liver. The green zinger is no exception when it comes to these benefits, and you can count on its advantages to not only enjoy balanced PH, but also several other upsides of this juice. Below is the process of making a tasty and healthy alkaline green juice.

Green Zinger Alkaline Juice

Yield

Servings for 2

Time

5 minutes

Ingredients

2 whole cucumbers

1 lemon

2 inch piece of Ginger

Handful of string beans

2 pears

1 to 2 tbsp. Chia seeds (added after making your juice)

Chia contains 50% Omega 3 acids, which enables slowing down the metabolism of sugars present in the pears to avoid incidences of insulin spikes. These seeds float to the top at first once added to your green juice.

You can thus use a cappuccino whisker to mix them for about one minute, until they full combine them with the juice. This enables Chia seeds absorb the juice, since they are highly hydrophilic. They will therefore absorb the liquid and expand to as large as 12 times their original size. They will also become softer and spread across the juice, mixing effectively.

And there you have your green zinger drink. With these ingredients handy, you can be sure to achieve a healthy drink that will not only help lower your alkaline levels, but also assist in other metabolic functions and organ development. What's more interesting about this juice is how easy it is to make, which makes it a favorite for many, and you can take advantage of the simple process and make yourself a healthy and tasty green juice as well.

If you are fond of taking acidic foods, you do not want to wait until the effects catch up with you, you can start to counter the results of your preferred diet before it turns against you. Now, there is no better way to ensure you are safe than grabbing a green drink.

16.

Magnesium Supplements; are they Necessary and Why

MAGNESIUM IS ONE OF the most vital minerals in the body. It may be taken for granted, but its lack can lead to grave effects. Therefore, it is important to take supplements if you are not getting enough of it from your diet. Here are several things you should know about magnesium and why it is so useful.

Symptoms of Magnesium Deficiency

If your magnesium levels drop below the optimum, you can experience complications from as simple as muscle weakness and cramps to complications like Alzheimer's disease. Other symptoms include damage in the liver and kidneys, cardiovascular diseases and hypertension, as well as severe PMS symptoms, insomnia, and osteoporosis. It is possible to experience mood swings and behavioral disorders, impotence, deficiency in Vitamin K, Vitamin B1, Calcium and potassium. If your magnesium levels drop, you are also bound to have recurrent fungal and bacterial infections from low nitric oxide as well as tooth cavities, multiple sclerosis, migraine headaches among others.

Causes of Low Magnesium

Some of the factors contributing to magnesium deficiency result from human activities and digestion failures. One of these causes is soil depletion, which in turn leads to low absorption of the component by crops. Digestive disorders also play a part in the problem, leading to malabsorption of magnesium and other nutrients. Increased use of antibiotics can also lead to this problem by damage to the digestive tract, which hinders magnesium absorption from foods.

Types of Common Supplements

Magnesium is present in foods, or as dietary supplements. It can also come from synthetically added to food products as well as in form of over-the-counter drugs like laxatives and antacids. The supplement comes in many forms.

Magnesium Citrate

This is magnesium combined with citric acid. It may have laxative effects if taken in large doses, but if used well, it helps with digestion and can prevent constipation.

Magnesium chelate

This type is naturally found in foods and is absorbed easily in the body. It is packed into amino acids for recovery of magnesium levels.

Magnesium Chloride

This is magnesium in oil form and can be applied on the skin. It is also useful for people with digestive disorders that make it difficult for magnesium to be absorbed from food. Athletes also find it handy for increasing endurance, energy and reducing muscle pain as well as for healing wounds and skin irritation.

Magnesium Threonate

This type can easily penetrate the mitochondrial membrane, hence making it easily absorbable. It is not as available, but with research, it will become more available in the future.

Magnesium Glycinate

This one is highly absorbable, and good for people with magnesium deficiency. It is also unlikely to cause laxative effect.

Magnesium is helpful for reducing such conditions as high blood sugar, metabolic syndrome, and diabetes among others. Researchers are also trying to figure out whether the introduction of magnesium supplements may be the solution for prevention of these diseases and disorders. Aging causes decreases in the ability to absorb adequate magnesium. This means that the elderly are in need for these supplements. There are many people facing the risk of chronic deficiency, whom may need to take these supplements as well.

17.

Top Five Advantages of Cinnamon to Your Health

CINNAMON HAS BEEN A favorite spice for many people over the years. Cinnamon spice has gained recognition the world over. It is delicious, but something more lies beneath its tasty nature. Science has found cinnamon worth of the credit for its healthy qualities. Here are few things about cinnamon that you should know.

Why cinnamon

One thing that makes cinnamon more than just a mere spice is a natural substance in the spice called cinnamaldehyde. This element is useful for its antibacterial and antifungal properties that qualify cinnamon as more than just a spice.

How to include it in Diet

You may need to take cinnamon to enjoy its positive side, but remember to take it easy on the spice. Cinnamon is toxic in large doses, which calls for prudence in its consumption. However, you can include just a pinch in your coffee, tea, or savory dishes, to get its aroma and flavor, as well as the health benefits it comes with. A 6 gram daily intake is advised, going for 6 weeks, and taking a rest before resuming.

Cinnamon comes in different types as cinnamon cassia (Chinese cinnamon), but you need to go for Cinnamon Verum, which is rich in essential components.

Benefits of Cinnamon

1. Packed with antioxidants

Cinnamon has antioxidants as polyphenols, which offer protection against body damage from oxidation by free radicals. According to a recent study, cinnamon is by far a reliable spice, which proves useful than most spices and superfoods like oregano and garlic. What is more interesting, this spice is powerful enough to be used as a food preservative.

2. Treatment for Alzheimer's and Parkinson's

These neurological diseases have proved incurable for some time, which calls for symptom treatment instead. The good news is that this treatment can be by an addition of cinnamon in your diet. The spice helps the performance of neurons and motor in people suffering from these diseases, helping reduce the impediment that comes with the symptoms, and allowing those suffering from the predicament live almost normal lives.

3. Reducing the risk of heart diseases

Cinnamon has proved a reliable remedy for heart diseases, a major cause of premature death globally. One gram of cinnamon daily helps blood markers for people suffering from type 2 diabetes, besides reducing LDL cholesterol and triglycerides, while maintaining HDL cholesterol levels. This spice can also help increase the good HDL cholesterol.

4. Lowering blood sugar

Cinnamon has a significant effect on blood sugar levels, reducing it by affecting insulin resistance and several other mechanisms. These include reducing the level of glucose entering the bloodstream by affecting digestive enzymes and slowing carbohydrates breakdown as a result. Cinnamon also contains a component that affects cells by imitating insulin, which improves glucose intake by the cells.

5. Anti-carcinogenic properties

Although limited to animal studies, a recent survey has revealed that cinnamon may have anti-carcinogenic effects. If the same applies to humans, then this spice is helpful in slowing growth of cancerous cells as well as killing them altogether.

18.

Top Five Benefits of Ginger

GINGER IS AMONG THE most popular spices in the world. The herb is also a major component when it comes to health issues. Ginger is tasty, but it also comes with significant benefits for your mental health as well as your body well being. However, there are ways in which you should use this herb since the upsides of proper use can be far reaching, but only when used prudently.

How to use ginger

Raw ginger is one of the many ways that people use this delicious spice. This way, a thumb size piece of ginger can be used in making vegetable juice at home.

Ginger oil is also a major potent form since it is high in gingerol, which makes it among the most efficient ways in which ginger can cater for medicinal purposes. Ginger can be used either internally or to rub on a sensitive area. Two to three drops can suffice for a therapeutic dose.

Ginger in powder form is also useful for this treatment, especially as a ground cooking spice. You can use it for pumpkin pie, chicken curry, or a ginger berry smoothie. If you take it in capsule form, go for 1,000 milligrams a day.

Ginger tea is yet a common remedy for nausea, stomach upset and for relaxing the body. In the case of inflammation, it is wise to take about two to three cups of ginger tea throughout the day.

Benefits of ginger

1. Treating nausea

Ginger is an effective remedy for nausea and vomiting, especially after surgery or chemotherapy treatment in case of cancer patients.

During pregnancy, ginger helps with nausea resulting from morning sickness. However, during pregnancy, consult with your doctor, since ginger may be unsafe if taken in large amounts in such condition. It is believed that excessive intake of the spice may lead to a miscarriage, although this is not scientifically proven yet.

2. Heart disease

If taken along with other super foods, regular use of ginger may come to your rescue against heart disease and stroke. Ginger, onion and garlic are useful anti-blood-clotting agents, and together they provide a reliable solution for heart attack and stroke alike.

3. Diabetes management

With its ability to increase insulin sensitivity, ginger has proved to be a reliable remedy for diabetes. According to research, ginger has been found to not only reverse diabetes but also prevent the disease and counter diabetes-related complications like diabetic retinopathy.

4. Treating chronic indigestion

Also known as dyspepsia, chronic indigestion symptoms include discomfort in the upper stomach and chronic pain. Indigestion results from the lack of timely removal of waste from the system. Ginger has shown excellent contribution in assisting emptying of the stomach in people with this problem, by reducing the time the process takes from 16 to 12 minutes.

5. Cancer prevention

Ginger has proved to be an alternative for treating several cancer types. Its anticancer properties come from its compound, 6-gingerol, which is substantial in raw ginger. Ginger extract reduces pro-inflammatory signaling, commonly found in the colon. Researchers also say that ginger can help with ovarian cancer, pancreatic cancer, and breast cancer.

20.
Top Six Daily Alkaline Foods for Good Health

WITH THE CURRENT STYLE of eating in the contemporary society, including alkaline food in your diet is inevitable to counter the effects of the widespread consumerist diet. Consumption of such food may necessitate moderation since excessive consumption can lead to complications too, but it is obvious that this is something you cannot overlook when planning your diet. If you do not know which alkalizing food you should consider, then here is a list of the top six foods that you can consider including in your diet for vibrant health.

1. Leafy greens

Greens have their fair share of reputation for being on top of the list as healthy and nutritious aspects of the everyday meal, and the case is not any different with the alkalizing function. Leafy greens like Swiss chard, kale, spinach and turnip greens are among the best in this field. Spinach is packed with vitamin K and folate, minerals and phytochemicals, fiber and antioxidants, which makes it able to boost vision and aid digestion.

2. Root vegetables

Roots too have something to offer, they also come with essential content that helps in balancing your diet. Talk of turnips, horseradish carrots, beets, and rutabaga. These roots do not require much more than a fast steaming for about 15 to 20 minutes, and they leave you feeling full and satisfied.

3. Garlic

If you are looking for alkaline-forming food, and an overall health ingredient to add to your diet, you should look no further, garlic has it all. Garlic also comes with several other benefits, including boosting immunity and cardiovascular health and reducing blood pressure as well as cleansing the liver and keeping diseases at bay.

4. Cayenne peppers

This pepper belongs to a group of peppers packed with enzymes that are useful in endocrine function. Cayenne ranks high in the list of the most alkalizing foods, and it also has its reputation for its antibacterial properties as well as being high in Vitamin A, which is essential in the pepper's effect against stress and illness.

5. Cruciferous vegetables

These veggies have already earned their widespread reputation for their healthy and tasty nature. If you like cabbage, broccoli, Brussels sprouts or cauliflower, then you should consider cruciferous vegetables. These veggies are an excellent way of making your diet a special treat for your body.

6. Lemon

Well, it's all about saving the best for last. Lemon may not be taken seriously as a useful fruit, but it is more than you might think. Lemon is actually among the most alkalizing foods, besides being a disinfectant in nature, which enables it to offer relief for wounds with hyperacidity and other conditions associated with viruses. Lemon is also a good remedy for flu, colds and cough, as well heartburn, and helps in energizing the liver and aids in detoxification.

21.

Ways of Reducing Acid Build Up

UNFOUNDED BELIEFS AND irregular eating patterns are to blame for the large rate of acidic people in the world today. It is for these very reasons that many have been religiously abiding to outlooks that lure them to consuming acidic foods which in turn complex their body functions. Such ill advice ends up rendering the consumers unhealthy and making regular visits to hospitals.

Our blood pH is the most vital part in our bodies. The blood pH acts as the closed circuit by which each solitary body part remains connected to the other. It is through the blood pH balance that the brain communicates amicably with other body parts. For healthy body operations, there must be consistent communication of different organs and cells in the body. When the pH is well balanced, the body as a whole is considered healthy.

When the body has high levels of alkaline, it is quite impossible for diseases and bacteria causing illnesses to prevail.

How to Achieve the Alkaline Blood pH

To avoid consumption of chemicals, pesticides, and other contaminants it is wise to carefully choose and consume organic food products only. One should also focus on eating alkaline foods only, foods such as fresh vegetables and fruits. Fresh fruits and vegetables diet are a great boost to sustenance of the blood's' pH balance.

Cut the daily intake of proteins such as from meats and cereal grains. Also try to avoid are all manners of refined sugars or flour. The maximum uptake of proteins per day should never exceed 40-50 grams since such foods contribute to acidity.

To have a balance of pH in your food, it is advisable to mix acidic products with alkaline ones. This assists in maintaining the blood pH balance create better body organ coordination. Ensure that you drink several glasses of water and apple cider mixture daily. Mix 2 tablespoons of apple cider vinegar against 8 ounces of water.

Notable Remedies for Acid-Alkali Balance

You could make a homemade remedy for the acidosis complications. By mixing half a teaspoon of sodium carbonate (baking powder) with two tablespoons of lemon juice, you come up with the best home remedy for acidosis. When the emanating fizz has settled, add to the mixture eight ounces of water and drain the mix at once. This mixture however may not go well with people with edema or hypertension conditions.

Bananas honey and lemons are known sources of high end calcium, magnesium and potassium. Consumption of such foods will help in maintaining balanced acid-alkaline levels. Lemon water assists the body system in creating an alkaline state against acidosis. Lemonade is effective in quelling nausea, overcome shock and relieve headaches. The light sour but refreshing taste of the lemonade should not be sweetened. The only thing that should be allowed to add is room temperature cooled water.

You should drink lots of water each day to assist your body in flushing out impurities. You should always ensure to drink half your weight every day. Consume digestive enzymes, such as bicarbonates, to assist your body's own production of enzymes. This ensures that your body is not overwhelmed with the production of digestive enzymes. If the pancreas may be overwhelmed it may cease to function properly.

22.

What mucus is and its scientific purpose

MUCUS IS A SLIMY BODILY fluid that tends to be stuffy and blocks the nasal cavity when someone has a cold. The fluid renders a discomfort and difficulty in normal breathing. Mucus is consistent of water, glycoprotein matter and other molecules. It is a viscous secretion that protects body organs and cavities.

Mucus is produced by and kept in all body cavities, not the nasal cavity only. Mucus is not particular to human beings; lots of other living creatures produce it too. For instance, the octopus employs mucus for keeping its burrow firm and prevents it from caving in. Earthworms use mucus for communication, while dolphins use mucus in clicking communicative noises. The bony fish ward off harmful and illness causing bacteria by covering its body in a shield of mucus.

The role of mucus in the human body

The slimy fluid that is mucus has several purposes in the human body. Mucus acts as a lubricant on the esophagus, easing the process of swallowing food. The lubrication ushers smooth passage of crushed food particles from the mouth to the stomach. In the stomach, mucus protects the linings from corrosive acids that trigger the digestive process.

In the nasal cavity, the mucus is an antiseptic fluid which flushes out intruders and protects the sinuses. Mucus also guards the nasal system from possible dangerous invaders. Mucus is at the frontline of bodily protection, using its non-Newtonian gel ability to trap and keep out even microscopic intruders.

Mucus is entirely effective in filtering the air we breathe in through the nose. This viscous fluid traps dust particles and other impurities such as smoke particles floating in the air, preventing them from entering the inner respiratory organs. Thus, mucus is an initial defensive mechanism in the body against all harmful bacteria.

The nose in particular produces approximately four cups of mucus on a daily basis. This slime is made up of mucin (a protein based lubricant) and water. Mucus has a variety of colors to adapt. It could be brown, yellow, brown, green or white. The color shade is dependent of some dead matter and cells stuck in the slime. White blood cells are responsible for the lighter shades of mucus. The mucin assists in keeping the trapped bacteria and other particles from clumping into biofilms.

What your mucus say about your health

When the nose tissue is inflamed, a red or brown pigmentation of the mucus will be visible. This will be an indication of red blood cells presence as a result of the tissue inflammation. A green pigmentation will in many cases indicate the requirement of antibiotics by the immune system.

There are two elements that build up the nasal mucus. One is a layer of fluid at the bottom known as the sol, which lends the mucus watery. Then there is the gel, which is sticky and traps the particles and bacteria. If the microscopic tentacles (cilia) in the nose are toggled, the mucus automatically gushes out to combat the intruder.

Excessive coughing and sneezing when one is sick are pointers of damaged cilia by the bacteria causing virus. The excessive coughs or sneezes occur as the body is struggling to rid of the excess mucus produced to assist in the healing of the damaged cilia.

23.

Effective Herbal Remedies for Inflammation

WHEN YOUR BODY IS INFLICTED by damage or injury, inflammation is the natural response that helps the body heal. Inflammation is thus a natural immune booster for tissue repairing or healing. If however the body starts chronically inflaming, it's a health concern. This is in turn is referred to as chronic inflammation. There are several causes of chronic inflammation including common modern stressors such as carrying extra weight, pollutions and food sensitivities.

Medically, chronic inflammation is tied to other life threatening diseases. These include Attention Deficit Disorder, heart diseases, diabetes cancer and the Alzheimer's disease. However contrary to mass belief, chronic inflammation is preventable and treatable. There are varieties of herbs that one can apply to reduce or keep inflammation at bay.

White willow bark as an inflammation remedy

The Egyptian and Roman empires widely used the white willow bark to treat inflammation and pain. Numerous studies have concluded that white willow has an effect similar to aspirin, only with bark less side effect as compared to aspirin.

Some herbal blends of white willow will be used to quell acute headaches and other secluded pain events. However, the recommended daily dose of white willow bark is 240mg for adults.

Cur cumin (found in Turmeric)

Cur cumin is the yellow pigmentation found in turmeric. It is believed to be an antioxidant that can be used to treat cancer. Turmeric can be added to foods, soups and curries in either its fresh form or as a ground powder. Fresh turmeric could also be added to fresh fruit and blended together, or even added directly to juices.

Especially the traditional Chinese and Ayurvedics globally use the turmeric (cur cumin) to treat infections, wounds and digestive disorders. Cur cumin can also be applied to meals as an additive.

Chili peppers in treating inflammation

There are infinite varieties of the capsaicin (pepper), but they share a common origin. The chili peppers are traceable to the tropics of America, where the Capsicum annum was first sighted. The chemical capsaicin retains the peppers hot effect and is present in all varieties of the chili. The capsaicin cures inflammation in the body.

The pepper can be used in all sorts of foods including desserts as a powder or fresh. Some supplements of capsaicin are mixed with other herbal elements to create natural anti-inflammatory purees.

Frankincense or Boswellia serrata

Frankincense is a resin of tree extracts. Resin is obtained from the Boswellia tree, a native of the Arabian Peninsula, India, Somalia and Ethiopia. Resin has pain-controlling effects, controls arthritis, and is anti-inflammatory in the human body. In modern medicine, frankincense is used to cure inflammatory and degenerative joint pains.

A mixture of Boswellia and cur cumin was used also in effectively treating osteoarthritis. A daily dosage of the frankincense resin is recommended in measures of between 300-500mg to cure or keep chronic inflammation in check.

Cloves for treating inflammation

During dental observation or treatment, the clove oil can be directly applied to the teeth gum. The oil is effective for alleviating toothaches. It is also an excellent pain controller, and acts fast upon application. Cloves have been in use to combating throat and mouth inflammation and as an expectorant for chest and cough reliefs.

They are also in use for treating hernia, diarrhea, nausea and bad breath. Cloves can be taken up by adding their powdered or dried whole flowers to foods and soups. The savory cloves are delicious in hot drinks as well as desserts too.

24.

Tips on Keeping a Healthy Vision with the Right Diet

VISION IS AT THE CENTER of every human activity, even to the meals we select and prepare. However, the most unfortunate thing is that vision health does not receive as much attention as it should. There is a lot you can do to maintain vision health, and the best means of all is by ensuring a diet that can keep your sight at its best. Here are few tips on having healthy vision.

Go for the right nutrients

Having the correct vision health takes time, but with the proper foods, you can live a life with healthier vision. One of the essential factors that make the difference is in the nutrient content of the foods you eat, and, more importantly, focusing on certain foods that will keep your vision on 20/20 form. Such nutrients as vitamin A are necessary for the retina, while mineral zinc and selenium also help in protecting this part of the eye. Additionally, fatty acids assist in moisturizing the eye.

What foods to choose

With all types of foods that many people like including in their diet list, one may think they have all they need to be healthy. And while carrot is thought to be the only essential food for visual health, much is left undiscovered, as there are various types of food that you need to choose as well. These include antioxidant green veggies, blueberries, eggs and acai that help your vision remain keen, now and as you age.

Leafy veggies like spinach and kale are high in lutein and zeaxanthin. These vegetables boost naturally occurring pigments inside the central part of the retina, helping reduce the risk of macular degeneration and cataracts. Additionally, broccoli, bright-colored fruits as grapes and collard greens are good for antioxidants, thus qualifying as an appropriate choice for vision health.

Veggies and fruits do the trick

Other foods like berries and citrus are high in vitamin C, which is also essential for preventing macular degeneration as well as cataracts. You also need to keep Brussels sprouts, papaya, green peppers and broccoli in your diet if you are to get sufficient supply of vitamin C. Almonds are also a recommendable aspect of bringing onboard, as it is packed with vitamin E, which is essential for maintaining muscular degeneration. If you can also get some pecans, vegetable oil, sunflower seeds, and a bit of wheat germ oil, which you can include in your salad, for a boost of this vitamin.

If you are on a consistent intake of these fruits and vegetables, you can be sure to have a fighting chance of maintaining your visions health. Alkaline diet is crucial now, count on it to ensure that your vision does not deteriorate as you age, which is the case with many people. Beta-carotene in carrots works wonders, but make sure to include these other useful constituents to keep your vision strong. What matters most is keeping veggies and fruits by your side, and taking it easy on saturated fats and sugars, which are not good for your vision.

25.

Tackling Numerous Myths Surrounding Cancer Treatment

CANCER IS ONE OF THOSE topics that would cause panic among many people all over the world. This disease has been a cause of concern for many families. This subject will be exhaustive before we understand it in detail since the myths associated with cancer make it difficult to separate reality about it from fiction. Here are some of the fictional myths about cancer.

Special diets can cure or prevent cancer

The first fallacy about cancer is centered on foods. Since cancerous cells are associated with thriving in acidic environments, glycolysis, a process of consumption of glucose blamed for cancer development. Although this was the suggestion of Otto Warburg in 1924, subsequent studies proved this is not the case. This is a result of the presence of cancer in the body. Therefore, this is an indicator that alkaline diet does not have any effect on cancer cells. Blood and the brain are responsible for the control of acidity in the body. Therefore, it is evident that sugar, acidity or alkalinity in the diet has nothing to do with the development of cancer or its treatment.

Homeopathy and other natural options can help

One proposed natural remedy for cancer is cannabis oil. This plant has assisted in clinics in managing pain and nausea for quite some time, and it is associated with being an effective cancer treatment. However, studies in the US and Cancer Research UK has shown that there is no evidence to support these claims. Homeopathy is the other commonly known remedy for this disease, but studies have proven that it does not have any significant effect more than placebo. The faith on this method could also be dangerously misleading thousands of patients.

Deodorants, artificial sweeteners, and cell phones are a red flag

Although deodorants have been associated with breast cancer, especially in the 1990s, studies have found no connection between the two. Artificial sweeteners have faced a similar fate, with many claims tagging them as neurotoxin poison. Nevertheless, studies on such sweeteners as aspartame, saccharin, sucralose, neotame, and acesulfame potassium have proved lack of evidence that supports such claims.

On another note, dubious claims have placed microwaves, cell phones, and power lines on the spot, blaming the electromagnetic radiation effects in these appliances on causing cancer. However, this has been a shear misconception, taking radiation for radioactivity. Long-term experimentation has proved that microwave energy used in most home appliances does not ionize DNA or damage cells (which could lead to cancer).

Cancer cure is available, but suppressed for profits

This is another general claim that there exists a cure for cancer, withheld through conspiracy for profit issues. However, the claim appears to cancel itself out, since with many cancer cases, who would hold back something for profits instead of going out there and selling it out?

What makes all of these theories about cancer and people who want to push alternative cures, diet plans and supplements are in their support. The hard reality for most people to comprehend; cancer remains a complex illness, comprising of diverse disease forms, and the proposed diets cannot cure it, nor is there a particular cure for this disease.

26.

Secret Treasures in Drinking Water

DEHYDRATION IS ONE of the most common complications that cause severe discomfort. If not addressed, dehydration will ultimately lead to loss of life of the affected person. This dangerous condition comes to effect when the body's water intake is lower than its output: the body loses more water than it receives.

The most effective preventive measure for dehydration is actually taking adequate water. People who thrive at high altitude areas and their arid areas counterparts are at a high risk of dehydration. Sports professionals are advised to regularly drink water since their bodies mostly engaged in water loss activities.

Water is the best fluid for your body

Other than combating dehydration, water has several other benefits to a human body. Aqua is recommended to those seeking to maintain weight loss or trim their body figure. For all who wish to maintain healthy weight, water is a mandatory consumption. This is because water has zero calories as compared to other dietary fluids recommended. Drinking water in place of soda or any other caloric beverage is more helpful in shedding the pounds off. Tooth rot, diabetes and obesity can be traced to caloric fluids, diet soda included. Water however is ultimately the healthiest drink one could ever have.

When your body is not adequately hydrated, it is easy for you to get fatigued. Fatigue is brought on by muscles getting sore, due to lack of hydrants. Drinking water alleviates fatigue and improves body performance. Weight loss during training or exercising can be coupled with dehydration.

Aqua is therapeutic to your skin and digestive process

Water is good for skin moisturizing and conditioning. A skin that is not well moisture will become flaky, tight and begin to crack. The skin will turn dry and is most likely to wrinkle in the absence of adequate water. It is however a tricky part in getting enough water to the skin since all other organs will have to be well hydrated before water gets to the skin. It is advisable that you apply a skin moisturizer as soon as you take a bath. Moisturizers assist in retaining skin moisture, as does drinking eight or more glasses of water each day.

Drinking enough water is a key point in maintaining perfect bowel function. In case there is a shortage of water in the digestive system, the colons skim water from the stool (refuse). This will in turn cause discomfort when you are relieving yourself. If the colon takes all the water from the stool, it causes constipation and consequent discomfort in the bowels too.

Clean bill of health

Drinking water has an array of merits for normal body operations. To achieve optimal body processes and healthy organs, you are required to maintain regular water intake. Numerous medical practitioners recommend that a normal and fully grown human being should drink eight or more glasses of water each day. This will greatly assist in ensuring that all body organs are adequately watered. Loss of water or lack of enough aqua fluid content in the body will lead to health complications.

27.

Lifesaving Apple Cider Vinegar Validations

NUMEROUS DISHES, DRESSINGS and sauces employ vinegar as an ingredient. Vinegar is associated with several other applications such as deodorizing, sanitizing and general cleaning. Of the several vinegar varieties available in the markets today, apple cider is the most popular in the kitchen.

Among other uses as mentioned above, apple cider vinegar is associated with effectively preventing or treating chronic diseases. Some of the ailments that apple cider vinegar is capable of handling include diabetes, cancer and cardiovascular conditions. Apple cider vinegar is consisted of body benefiting bacteria, high level proteins and enzymes.

The Expansive uses of Apple Cider Vinegar

Vinegar has an acidic component that is capable of killing or limiting the growth of bacteria. It is for this reason that apple cider is widely used as a disinfectant. It is also applied as a food preservative and fungicide. Its ability to control bacterial growth fames apple cider vinegar as a food preservative. Foods preserved with this vinegar have a shelf life extension of up to a year. All pickle processed foods have vinegar as a preservative.

Popular shampoos and hair products cause a particular build up in the hair after some duration of use. This product buildup is removable through using apple cider vinegar. Apple cider vinegar leaves the hair untangled and with a shiny effect. The vinegar should however be mixed with equal ratios of water before use and left to linger on the hair a short while before rinsing. An acid in the vinegar also controls Malassezia and should thus be applied to rid of dandruff.

Vinegar has been proven by medical practitioners as to normalize blood sugars. It is effective in controlling blood sugar of people with pre-diabetic and diabetic conditions. Thus a diet consistent of apple cider vinegar is recommendable. However diabetic people should always consult their medical care provider before starting or adding their vinegar consumption. This is done to exempt any risky antagonism with prescribed diabetic medication. Consequently apple cider vinegar has been applied to quell cholesterol issues and high blood pressure and triglycerides.

Vinegar as a Holistic Cancer Combatant

Apple cider vinegar is respected and validated as a cancer cell combatant. Laboratory assessment has confirmed the fact that apple cider is capable of killing or slowing the growth of cancerous cells in the body. Vinegar is an exceptional blood pH acid balancing agent, a thing that many scientists have evaluated as a means of limiting cancer cell development.

An Apple cider meal can also be combined with carbohydrate based meals for people wishing to shed off weight. Apple cider vinegar triggers a satisfactory feeling in the belly, thus reducing extravagant consumption. Apple cider vinegar proceeds to flatten the belly fat and evening the waist circumference. It also has a confirmed weight loss yardstick of two pounds every month in daily usage.

As a blood sugar stabilizer, apple cider vinegar acts in the similar mandate as some common diabetic pills only with lesser side effects. Significant blood glucose sensitivity can be fully optimized by complementing every possible meal with apple cider vinegar. This proves that apple cider vinegar, a common kitchen ingredient, has multiple lifesaving abilities.

28.

Extra Health Packed in Alkaline Water

HEALTH EXPERTS CLAIM that alkaline water has multiple advantages to the human body. Alkaline water is capable of slowing aging and preventing chronic ailments such as cancer, infertility, increases energy levels and regulates body pH balance.

Alkaline is available as packaged in bottled water in the market shelves. Hydration is healthy to your body's metabolism and water is calorie free. Pure water has a pH scale of 7, set in the middle of the alkali-acid measurement which runs from 1 to 14. A liquid situated at the point 1 is regarded as highly acidic while one at 14 is purely basic (alkaline). Alkalized water has a higher pH than ordinary water at 9.5.

At an approximation of 7.4 human blood levels are somewhat alkaline, and these levels should be highly maintained. Other body organs have a variance in their ph. level; the stomach for instance must remain quite acidic to conduct normal digestion. Your body is massive 80% water and must be kept in regular check to maintain the recommended pH balance for optimal health.

Maintaining the pH Balance

If pH balance in your body is not adequately maintained, the body reaches out to the bones to source the needed minerals to neutralize the acidity in excess. High acidosis will lead to anxiety, diarrhea, possible loss of sight and impaired immunity. All the above complications can be kept in check by drinking alkaline based fluids.

Drinking alkaline water for some 3 to 6 months greatly assists in lowering blood pressure, blood glucose and cholesterol levels in the human body. Alkaline water also neutralizes the levels of pepsin and stomach acid therefore allowing for treatment of acid reflux. The intake of alkalized water amongst senior citizens is helpful in efficiently curbing dementia and memory lapse.

When compared to tap water, mineral based alkaline water improves hydration and a balance in the acid-alkali status in the human body. Natural alkaline water gathers its minerals from the rocks as it runs down stream. Multiple minerals such as zinc, potassium, magnesium among others are tucked in the environments that envelope streams. Run offs carry the minerals to the rivers and streams settling these at the rock beds. When you consume from stream water and consume, one can be sure that the stream water is basically alkalized.

Homemade Alkalized Water

Another form of alkalized water is homemade with the assistance of water ionizing equipment. There are several manufacturers who produce and market the ionizing machine, but they may not be cost friendly. The machine simply utilizes a chemical procedure called electrolysis, where the water molecules are electrocuted for separation thus making them more basic or acidic.

Adding a squeeze of an alkaline based fruit such as lemon to your water also turns the water into base. Lemon juice and lime are practically acidic but they carry certain composites capable of altering the water status, from acidic to alkaline. You can also use pH drops in your water and make it more alkaline.

Excess consumption of alkaline water is however discouraged especially for people with pre-existing kidney complications. This is because the extra minerals could end up hurting your kidneys since they are not entirely soluble with a kidney malfunction. It is however necessary to note that alkaline water is ultimately good for optimal body health.

29.

Eating Smart: Zinc keeps away Infections

ZINC IS WIDELY NEEDED in all body parts. It assists in the improvement of the body's immune system. The most vital roles that zinc plays in the body include: breaking down carbohydrates, cell division, cell growth and healing wounds or tissue breakages. Zinc also improves smell and taste senses.

Zinc is a metal vital in element of trace. It is important to note that everyone is required to consume small amounts of zinc daily. This assists in maintaining healthy body processes and optimal body organ operations.

Zinc has a variety of therapeutic benefits in the body. It is a great booster in the body's immunity in fighting chronic diseases such as cancer. Zinc also assists in combating inflammation, and vital in reversing cardiovascular conditions. This food additive also helps in balancing, repairing and production of hormones. Zinc is a major assistant to all immune systems and quells indigestion.

Aging is slower within the body tissues as its effects are reduced by zinc. This means that zinc is anti-oxidant that is capable of fighting free radical tissue damages. Because of its role in hormonal balance, any deficiency or lack of zinc may cause diabetes and infertility.

One becomes more susceptible to diseases and illnesses when their zinc levels are waning. Zinc is so vital that its deficiency will hinder the development of; the skeletal and immune systems, central nervous system, hormonal production, gastrointestinal, loss of water (integumentary dehydration), and a healthy reproductive system.

Symptoms of zinc deficiency

Some of the common symptoms of zinc deficiency deposits include fatigue, often getting sickly, and poor concentration. A loss of appetite, hair loss, loss of taste or smell, weight gain or loss and nerve dysfunction is also major pointers of zinc deficiency. Zinc helps in alleviating inflammation and oxidative stress, both of which are associated with chronic diseases such as heart conditions and cancers.

Most refined or processed foods in the market shelves do not contain zinc. Polished white rice and refined flour and sugar will be laden with energy, but lack essential micronutrients including zinc. Zinc is responsible for regulating the protein concentration in our bodies. Deficiency in zinc thus compromises the ability for tissue repair in our DNA.

Foods High in Zinc Concentration

There are high levels of zinc deposits in a number of foods, especially products high in protein. Ideally the concentration of zinc in raw, unpasteurized dairy products and organic milk is quite recommendable. Zinc traces are also high in sea foods high quality organic meats and animal proteins.

Legumes and grains also contain zinc, while particular processed cereals have zinc added to provide all around healthy meals. However these types of zinc are hard to absorb by the body since they contain phytates, an anti-nutrient that hinders zinc absorption.

High intake of carbohydrates, such as found in legumes and grains is a major culprit of the causes of zinc deficiency. This is because the carbohydrates replace the high protein sources making it hard for the digestive system to absorb the small amount of zinc. Vegetarians are also at a high risk of zinc deficiencies, because their choice of foods lack source of high end proteins. Consumption of animal products and meats is thus highly recommended. Although some vegetables contain zinc for example; asparagus or Brussel sprouts, green beans, corn, potatoes, and pumpkin. Avocados also have a significant amount of zinc.

30.

Ancient Egyptian Herbs for Holistic Healing

ARCHEOLOGISTS COMBING through ancient Egyptian tombs, underground temples and burial sites have unearthed extensive documents and scrolls detailing aged medicinal records. The scrolls such as the London Medical Papyrus, the Edwin Smith Papyrus, the Ebers Papyrus and the Hearst Papyrus also contain the earliest known records of tumors. The scrolls are proof of a high dependency on herbs in the ancient Egyptian empires.

To cure bronchial-pulmonary issues and asthma, the Egyptians would consume raw garlic and onions. The garlic and onions were also consumed raw as a sign of endurance. Fresh cloves of garlic were peeled, mashed and mixed with water and vinegar. The mixture would then be used for rinsing toothaches and sore throats. There is also information on usage of oral medicines. The medicines were made by steeping the herbs in wine. The herbs were all organic without any chemical or pesticide inducement. Egyptians had documented the use of an array of herbs such as frankincense, aloe, thyme, cassia and myrrh.

Medicinal ointments and their significance

Honey was used to produce medicinal ointments and medicines in fair share. Honey was also extensively applied as a natural antibiotic. The first formal recognition of the use of honey as a medicinal substance can be traced to the Egyptian dynasty. Temples unveiled contain hieroglyphics depicting the processes by which workers harvested honey. Indeed the renowned hive smoking is well illustrated on the walls of the dug-out archeological temples.

Historical facts reveal that the bee was a regarded with high respect, such that even one Pharaoh's title was the Bee King. Egyptian medicine is among the oldest documented and these remained relevant, consistent and very advanced up until the Persian invasion. Historians claim that the Egyptians were more skilled in the art of medicine more than any other field of expertise.

Modern medicine largely borrows from the Egyptian medical documents, more so the scroll christened the Edwin Smith Papyrus. Minerals, fruits, animal products and fats, herbs and vegetables were commonly employed to treat distinct ailments. The Ebers Papyrus on the other hand is the most voluminous of all Egyptian medical scrolls. Also in the papyrus is a detailed heart treatment practice, one recognizing the heart as the epicenter of the human body.

Herbs popular with ancient Egyptian medicines

Dementia, depression and mental disorders were also addressed in the ancient Egyptian medicine practice. Other treatments included the cure of tumors, intestinal complications and exemption of parasites, eyes and skin conditions among others. It is without doubt that the Egyptian healers were well versed in the human anatomy, proper hygiene and organic based medicines.

For instance, Persian henna was utilized against hair loss or paranormal balding. There was a particular manner of straining select roots with water to produce alkaloids. The alkaloids were drunk to force tapeworms relent their hold on the digestive system. Coriander was drunk as an herbal tea to cure kidney complications including cystitis.

Onions were recommended for those with heart conditions, and to prevent and cure common colds. Turmeric was directly used on open wounds and would accelerate healing. Thyme would be administered as a pain reliever.

31.

Affirmative Ways to Controlling and Reversing Diabetes

BASED ON MODERN EATING habits and lifestyles, one out of every three infants will struggle with diabetes in later stages of their lives. Scientific based projections state that diabetes affects approximately over a quarter billion people globally. Chronic diseases such as cancer, impotence, loss of sight, cardiovascular complexities, stroke and brain damage and limb amputations are all induced by diabetes. Two of three diabetics will die of heart attacks or stroke, yet it is possible to control and cure diabetes.

Diabetes is essentially of two major types, namely type 1 and type 2. Type 1 diabetes is brought on by the failure of the pancreas to produce insulin. Type 2 - diabetes is caused by abnormal reaction of the body to the insulin produced. Here the body's metabolism is unable to absorb glucose needed for effective processes. Diabetes is the body's inability converting blood sugar to requisite energy.

Managing Diabetes is Effortless in the Mind

Although diabetes is largely a nutritional deficiency it is also heavily dependent on the emotional aspect involved. Studies have shown that an individual's stress and experiences greatly contribute to their metabolism processes. Stress management, meaningful work and body exercise coupled with the immediate everyday environment will affect thought processes. Thus a person's community engagement will determine their body's emotional load and metabolism (acid production).

The kind of food a person consumes also point into the amounts of acid their body produces. If one is not observant of balancing their blood's pH levels via consumption of alkali-acid food, they will definitely end up producing too much metabolic acid. If the diet falls short of necessary minerals over years, then the alkali reservoirs of the body are depleted thus risking the production of more acid than required. Such alkali deficiencies will result to intracellular acidosis which in turn prevents the cells ability to rid of or refuse. To thus manage the diabetic situation effectively one is required to cautiously assess their diet.

Too much of fat and protein consumption than demanded by the body will result in a reduction of dietary fiber and vital nutrients. This leads to food over stuffing yet malnutrition, meaning that you are too full of mere refuse. Continued abuse of diet will in turn result to high cholesterol, high blood pressure and consequent diabetes. Consumption of dietary fiber, dense nutrition and required supplements is recommended as well as eating biodynamic (organic) foods.

Optimal Dieting against Diabetes

Acidic diets are tied to cardio-metabolic risks which will in turn lead to prediabetes. Elevated triglycerides, visceral obesity and high blood sugar are indicators doctors' today track in determining insulin resistance diabetes. The most intriguing fact is that the above outlined pointers are also similarly applied in evaluating cancer. They are considered risk factors for cancer observation.

With increased acidity, there is heightened risk of kidneys and urinary tract damage. This is brought about by lack of crucial minerals such as zinc, potassium and magnesium. Such minerals are required to buffer and safely rid of excess acids from the body. If there is a deficit in these vital minerals, there must be a system in check and if necessary induce supplements of the minerals. This way you keep acidosis and diabetes at bay.

32.

Benefits of Reducing Red Meat Consumption

ALTHOUGH RED MEAT IS a tasty favorite for many, it comes with its downsides. However, it is also worth noting that at the same time, there are shortcomings that will come with avoiding eating this kind of meat, as it has a fair share of nutrients too. These differences are significant, and depend on your health requirements or personal preference. Here are 11 things that happen if you stop eating red meat.

1. Weight loss

Since Red meat is packed with calories, cutting back its regular consumption could mean shedding a few pounds. This type of meat provides more proteins than required, with three-ounce serving having almost 170 calories, while a similar portion of beans have about 100 calories. Therefore, it could be wise avoiding it and moving to restore the protein loss by using less-calorie sources.

2. You can reduce body acid

PH balance is vital for healthy living, but the unfortunate reality is that most of the today's diets are acid-forming foods. Red meat, coffee, white flour, and soda are part of this class. This increase in acid in the body results in diseases, stress, and lack of sleep as well as leaving you vulnerable to diabetes and cancer among other grave illnesses. If you reduce your red meat consumption, this will make a significant impact in keeping high acid levels at bay.

3. You start feeling less bloated

Red meat can cause constipation in some people, since the body digests this food slowly, causing possible cases of gas and abdominal pain. This type of food can also lead to indigestion, which can cause feelings of bloating. Keeping red meat in check and embracing foods high in fiber can help reduce this problem significantly. A study has confirmed that vegetarians have lower cases of inflammation as compared to meat enthusiasts.

4. Possible skin improvement

Healthy skin is achieved by taking adequate vitamins like A, C and E that reduce radicals affecting the skin. While constipation from red meat can cause dull complexion and compromise skin health, avoiding it altogether can offer you healthier skin as well as other major organs like liver and kidneys benefits.

5. Lower cholesterol levels

Red meat is notorious for its saturated fat content, which is a leading cause of high cholesterol. Therefore, since cholesterol level should be maintained at 7% per day to reduce the risk of plaque building up in arteries and causing diseases, taking it slow on red meat helps prevent this menace.

6. Reduced risk of some types of cancers

Among the various benefits of keeping red meat at bay is a reduction in the risk of bowel, and colon cancers. This reduction works by avoiding the high saturated fat red meat, which leads to inflammation in the body responsible for cancer development. Besides studies has found that heme, which is a compound in meat that gives it the red color, is capable of being carcinogenic, not to mention nitrates and preservatives in processed meat that can also contribute to cancer.

7. Reduced risk for other diseases

Red meat saturated fat has also been linked with high risk of obesity, cardiovascular diseases, and diabetes. Red meat can also cause carnitine that can lead to Trimethylamine-N-oxide (TMAO). Besides, meat lovers are also at high risk for conditions like Alzheimer's disease, which you can avoid by reducing red meat on your diet list.

8. More energy

According to scientific studies, red meat consumption can trigger high levels of estrogen that causes hormonal balance, leading to a plunge in energy. The longer it takes to digest this meat the faster it leads to energy deficiency, as well as possibilities of poor absorption leading to irritable bowel syndrome, poor nutritional balance, and acid reflux among other problems.

9. Advantage to the environment

Benefits of taking it slow on red meat not only manifest in your body but also in the environment alike. Gathering animals for meat takes up tremendous amounts of energy, water, land, food and cause animal suffering as well, reducing red meat consumption will provide environmental benefits.

10. Avoid unnecessary protein

You may be consuming red meat for protein, which is the primary contribution it adds to your serving, but the question is actually how much protein you need altogether. It is possible that, since the need for proteins depends on factors like age, activity, and size, it is worth understanding the need for this nutrient. If you do not need that much of it, then you can reduce consumption if possible.

11. Lack of some nutrients

As much as red meat may be condemned for its downsides, it does come with some positive input. This meat offers a considerable amount of nutrients that you may need to consider if you stop taking it and do not consume any supplements. These include vitamin B12, B, and mineral Iron.

There is a lot that you can change by keeping red meat consumption under check. This is helpful for your body and the environment at large.

33.

Normal Weight Body Types Also More Prone to Diabetes

ONE OF THE MAJOR RISKS to being affected by Type 2 diabetes is when you are overweight or obese, that's no fallacy. However detailed studies have shown even lean people are in danger of acquiring diabetes. Such is probable if your lifestyle choices are somewhat unhealthy: choices such as smoking, how frequent you exercise are mixtures for disaster on your health.

Your favorite beverage could also lead to diabetes, contemporary investigation have viewed drinks as risk factors for diabetes too. If you are in the habit of drinking even a single sweetened drink or sugary beverage on a daily basis, you are at high risk of acquiring diabetes in a decade. People who never consume sugary drinks are clearly exempted of such risks, the studies have indicated.

Even lean or medium weight body types are at the risk of diabetes if they consume sugary drinks on a daily basis. The conclusion of several studies show that the continuous drinking of sweetened drinks (sweet tea included) will definitely bridge you and Type 2 diabetes.

The ties between diabetes and sugary beverages are solidified by the ability of medical researchers in explaining how excess sugar overwhelms the endocrine system. Artificially sweetened drinks are directly linked as notable causes of diabetes; such conclusion was not arrived at when analyzing fruit juices. All sweet drinks are blacklisted for people who want to control diabetes.

Potentially, numerous diabetes cases can be brought under check if only people were willing to change their day to day lifestyles. Not even the so called diet beverages are safe, although many overweight and obese people will at times turn to the diet drinks due to other health concerns. Beverage manufacturing enterprises are however opposed to these findings daring the researchers to show tangible evidence between the sugary drinks and their alleged chronic disease triggers.

Excess food consumption and diabetes

These studies are however based on keen observation and scientific interpretation of subjects and their routine in terms of food consumption and resulting outcomes over a specified time length. Consumption of excess food of any kind (sugar included) consequence to overweight, and the inevitable obesity spirals down to diabetes.

Increased sugar consumption by people even of normal weight will ultimately link to diabetes hitting higher among the populations. Excessive soft drink consumption also causes another sugar associated health concern known as Latent Autoimmune Diabetes in Adults (lada), a condition that exhibits signs and symptoms evidenced by both the Type 1 and Type 2 diabetic conditions. Lada is fairly uncommon today but there are concerns that the condition could escalate to bigger margins in the future.

Type 1 diabetes disease wipes out all insulin developing cells in the pancreas, while the Type 2 diabetes alters the body's response towards the insulin produced. A mixture of the two complications is evidently of even dire effects and the more reason you are urged to eliminate sugary foods and drinks. One outstanding pointer to diabetes is increased thirst, this indicating a possibility of diabetes first affecting a person and they in turn result to overconsumption of sugary drinks.

34.

Type 2 Diabetes: Causes and Measures

DIABETES IS A CHRONIC and life threatening disease that has seen rapid growth in numbers of those affected. Approximately, diabetes affects three times more people today than a decade ago. Diabetes is a lifestyle disease brought about by unhealthy consumption of sugars and high fructose corn syrup, especially those associated with processed foods. Diabetes is caused by the body's inability to generate insulin or use the insulin produced. Insulin is a body hormone that assists in transforming sugar (glucose) in the blood to energy in cells.

There two types of diabetes, namely juvenile diabetes (also referred to as type 1 diabetes), which accounts to about 5% of all diabetes cases. This occurs when the body is unable to produce the hormone insulin. There are no documented accounts of a means of preventing this type of diabetes.

The second type of diabetes (type 2 diabetes) is most common and is preventable but overwhelmingly represents 95% of all diabetes cases in the world. It commences with the body's inability to use insulin, over time however the pancreas ultimately is unable to make any insulin whatsoever. This results in the inability of the body to balance its blood sugar levels.

When the blood sugar levels are high but do not qualify to be categorized as diabetes, the resulting condition is known as prediabetes. This condition is also referred to as impaired fasting glucose or impaired glucose tolerance. People with prediabetes are more likely to develop Type 2 diabetes and heart disease.

If not checked effectively within early stages, 35% of people with impaired glucose intolerance will graduate to the Type 2 diabetes in five years. The remaining 65% will gradually creep into Type 2 diabetes in their life cycle.

Sugar spiked beverages are costly

One of the major drivers of Type 2 diabetes is liquid sugar, a sugar added to beverages as a sweetener. As the consumption of sugary beverages rises, so does the risk of acquiring Type 2 diabetes. The sugary beverages are the biggest culprit for their calories and sugars are ingested in fluid form. Liquid sugar is rapidly absorbed in to the body and the excess glucose spikes the insulin in a manner that it is unable to separate the blood sugar in the cells. The excess sugar ultimately ends up into fat in the liver, a straight channel to Type 2 diabetes.

A drink or two of extra sweetened beverages in a day has an increment of Type 2 diabetes risk by over 25%. In approximation, Type 2 diabetes and heart disease are both set at higher probability in people who continuously drink sugary drinks every day for a half year. Those who drink a lot of the sweetened beverages thrive in undiagnosed diabetic vacuum. People who have been diagnosed of diabetes are cautious when consuming the sweetened drinks.

Without proper management and careful considerations, diabetes will lead to blindness, heart attacks, stroke, amputations, and kidney failure and at the extremes death. The cost of managing diabetes is high and dear to both the individual and the community. The complications brought about by diabetes greatly influence the expenditures in terms of medication and hospital stays.

35.

Things You Should Know about Pineapple Water

Pineapple water has claimed its fair share of credit for outstanding benefits over the years. From antioxidant protection to essential minerals and vitamins to protecting the liver, this fruit is just incredible. Here are ideas about making this tasty and advantageous drink for yourself or your family, as well as some of its benefits.

PINEAPPLE HAS NUTRIENTS like Vitamin C, copper, manganese and folate. Besides, this fruit is renowned for its bromelain content, which has several benefits to the body as well.

How to make pineapple water

Start by cutting pineapple chunks, remove the rind, and then add them to a jug full of chilled water and ice.

Leave the water to chill in a fridge for several hours so that the pineapple can infuse the water.

Alternatively, when making pineapple-infused water, you can cut the fruit in half, remove and retain the rind. Then bring a liter of water to a boil, cut your pineapple into chunks and toss them into the boiling water. You can then add your rind to enhance the flavor. Keep boiling for about 20 minutes, and then let the mixture cool for about 15 minutes before straining the liquid into a pitcher and placing the mixture into the refrigerator to cool.

If you wish, you can add several other fresh and healthy ingredients like a cinnamon stick or a rosemary twig to your pineapple water to boost the content.

Benefits

• Fights inflammation

If there is one thing pineapple is known for is its fight against inflammation due to its rich content of bromelain and enzyme. Pineapple juice also helps flush out the liver and intestines, leaving you feeling less bloated. Bromelain destroys toxins that cause pain, fluid retention, edema and attack tissues. The drink also helps in relieving arthritis and joint pains from sports.

• Essential for weight loss

If you are looking into reducing your body weight, you will find the answer in daily consumption of pineapple water. With rich fiber content, this drink takes a long process to be break down, keeping you feeling great and off foods that may pump sugars and fats into your system. This also helps if you are trying to keep sugar cravings at bay as well. What's more important, a pineapple water detox can help get rid of impurities and several pounds.

• High in Vitamin C

This water-soluble antioxidant in pineapple water is ideal for fighting free radicals. These radicals can damage cells, promote plaque building up in arteries and cause heart diseases, and cause spasm in airway leading to an asthma attack. There's also a possibility of attacking colon cells and cause colon cancer, joint pain, rheumatoid arthritis and osteoarthritis among other complications.

• Boosts energy production

If you have pineapple water by your side, you can be able to increase energy production in mitochondria, thanks to its mineral manganese. It also has thiamin and B vitamin, which are essential for energy production.

Pineapple water gives you every reason to try it, and the best part is that you can never go wrong with this drink. It delivers when it comes to health benefits and other advantages as well. Go ahead, have this tasty juice, and see what it can do.

36.

The Hazards of Soybean Oil

ONE OF THE MOST DANGEROUS aspects of most diets is soybean oil, especially when you consume the hydrogenated one. This oil comes with its fair share of Trans fat, which makes it a hazard, not to mention other risks that the soy itself poses. Here are several things you need to watch out for the next time you consider using soybean oil.

How to hydrogenate and why

Hydrogenation is inducing hydrogen gas into the oil under high pressure, meant to prolong the oil's shelf life. This process also stabilizes the oil and raises its melting point, making it ideal for use in different food processing types that employ the use of high temperatures. However, if the oil is not "fully hydrogenated" then it contains the dreadful Trans fats that you do not want on your table. Besides, neither is the fully hydrogenated one safe as well.

Hazards of the Trans fat

These fats are known to cause chronic problems like asthma, cancer, autoimmune disease, obesity and bone degeneration. It also causes diabetes, heart diseases, and increasing the risk of cardiac arrest in women with coronary heart disease. Other issues include decreased immunity, a rise in blood levels, and reproductive problems from interfering with enzymes responsible for the production of sex hormones.

Shortcomings of Soybeans

It is not as if the soybean itself does not come with given complications. Especially when you combine the hydrogenated GE soybean oil, then you are headed for the worse. Soybeans contain substantial amount of omega-6 fat, which when highly processed, it becomes damaged, and thus you end up consuming a lot of it in your diet. This fat can cause chronic inflammation, capable of causing almost all chronic diseases.

Organic soybean oil

Natural soy may sound like the ultimate choice for you, but this may not be the ideal option yet. These beans can lead to:

Phytic acid- this acid is responsible for blocking the absorption of such minerals like magnesium, zinc, iron, and magnesium since phylates bind to metal ions.

Hemagglutinin- this substance causes clumping of your red blood cells together leading to clotting and preventing absorption and distribution of oxygen to tissues.

Goitrogen- this is found in unfermented soy, whether organic or not, and it blocks synthesis of thyroid hormones, thus interfering with the metabolism of iodine and thyroid function.

Natural toxins- such anti-natural factors as soya toxin, protease inhibitors, saponins, and oxalates, in soy, interfere with enzymes that help in digestion, which can be fatal for your health.

Genetically Engineered Soybean oil

Animal studies have also put this type of oil in the conversation, with its causes for increased infertility rates with each and any generation, with high infant mortality rate at second generation and the effects utterly devastating by the third generation.

Glycophytes in GE Soybeans

The residue level in GE soybeans is toxic, at 17 mg/kg. This residue has been associated with malformations in frog and chicken, with the worst effects on plants and passing all the way to humans. This underrated poison is applied to crops and is eaten in diet, affecting the gut, and possibly decimating your beneficial bacteria. With the good and bad bacteria ratio in your gut determining your immunity wellbeing, you can be at risk if these levels are altered. This substance also causes DNA damage, cancer, and toxicity (neurotoxicity, developmental and reproductive).

These harmful fats can take a toll on your health with time, and the best thing to do is keep them at bay. You can do this by just reducing or avoiding processed foods. You can instead try eating raw fats, cooking with coconut oil, olive oil, and or using organic butter.

37.

Sugar – The Hidden Poison

SUGAR IS USED BY NUMEROUS households for multiple reasons every day. It is a common sweetener applied in different recipes and as an additive. The problem with sugar is that it is highly addictive, and when used without much consideration, sugar leads to chronic illnesses. Almost every person craves for a taste of sugar, oblivious of its fatal consequences.

When we eat too much sugar, the reward centers in our neural systems become over stimulated leading to addiction. If you consume excess sugar, the reward centers open up realizing large amounts of dopamine. Dopamine is a feel good enzyme in the human body, it is the one responsible for the ecstatic feeling we have after eating sugar. Like drugs, sugar is addictive and equally deadly. People struggling with sugar cut backs go through unmatched torments; it is extremely difficult to recover from sugar addiction.

Sugar is a poison at your table

Often consumption of high sugar foods lead to the development of a specific tolerance that in turn demands more sugar to gain the dopamine rewards as explained overleaf. Within certain durations, you develop an addiction to the sugar via the over stimulation of the reward centers, simply because we are having more sugar based on the want to feel good. The amount of control with which sugar overrides your brain is similar to that of cocaine and heroin, sugar should thus be taken with top notch caution.

It is entirely intriguing to learn that more people get hooked to sugar daily. Studies recommend that men should not exceed nine teaspoons of sugar a day. Women on the other hand are limited to six teaspoons of sugar each day. Many however consume double the amount, most of which is in sodas and fruit juices. It is not mere coincidence that the two food s also happens to be the leading sources of excess calories in your body presently.

There are two common types of sugars; the natural and the added sugar. Natural sugar is sourced among fresh fruits and some vegetables; the added sugar is industrial manufactured. Added sugar has zero nutritional value and no vital vitamins, proteins or minerals that your body requires. It is also the most dangerous sugar and its toxicity is beyond normal. Added sugar has severe effects to your metabolism and triggers several chronic diseases.

Health complexities tied to sugar

Excess sugar in your system is a sure bet for inflammation and other health complexities. There are studies which have actually linked sugar consumption as a major cause for breast cancer. Obesity and cardiovascular diseases are also tied to excess sugar uptake.

Most of the added sugar you consume is well hidden in the processed foods under some popular name. Titles such as fructose, glucose, lactose, dextrose or maltose are mere cover up names for processed sugar. One must be very keen when purchasing their food so as to look out for the amount of food you consume.

If you are to consume sugar, it is only cautious and healthy to ensure that it is directly from fresh fruits. This way you are ensured of safe and the amount of sugar you take is minimal. However fruits too are somewhat high in sugars and you should thus not overeat.

38.

Skin and hair alkaline detox salad

THIS DELICIOUS SUMMER salad will have your skin glowing and have your hair shiny in no time. The food is effective in soothing inflammation while keeping your scalp and skin healthy. If you are struggling with skin redness, acne, rosacea, hair loss and baldness, this alkaline diet will work miracles for you. Conventional skin remedies do not work as you would expect in controlling aging effects on hair and skin. You may slather numerous chemicals in trying to sort out your skin and hair yet you may not acquire desired effects.

The problems keep on resurfacing because you are not treating the root causes of the issue. Most of the skin and hair malfunctions are as a result of diet deficiencies. Alkaline diets are the best way to treating your skin conditions from the inside out.

Skin and hair detox salad

4 servings

Dry mixture Ingredients

- 4 tablespoons flax seeds
- 4 tablespoons pumpkin seeds
- 2 tablespoons poppy seeds
- 1 teaspoon sea salt
- ½ tablespoon red pepper chili

Directions

In a sizeable mixing bowl, thoroughly mix the seeds, sea salt and dried chili and put aside.

Ingredients for the salad

- 4 finely grated carrots

- ½ finely chopped or grated celery root
- 1 fennel well sliced
- 2 cups arugula
- 2 cups finely sliced green cabbage
- 2 cups finely sliced red cabbage
- 1 avocado cubed
- Large handful of sprouts (broccoli or alfalfa)
- 8 tablespoons of extra virgin olive oil
- 1 finely sliced tomato (optional)

Directions

Combine the arugula with the celery, carrots, zucchini, fennel and the cabbage after you have finely chopped or grated.

Add the prepared dry mix you had set aside and thoroughly mix.

Share the salad in small serving bowls for the individuals. Dress the servings with sprouts and cubed avocado.

Sprinkle the salad with the extra virgin oil.

Add some more sea salt for tasting before tabling the healthy alkaline dish.

Regular yet best foods for your skin

Your skin requires regular hydration to remain moist and shiny. The foods you take are essential hydrants for your whole body. Products such as hemp seeds, chia, flax, salmon, avocado and coconuts contain high levels of fatty acids which work wonders in nourishing hair and skins.

Dark and leafy green vegetables assist in optimizing your digestive system by cleaning out harmful toxins and unwanted hormones that build up on the scalp if not kept in check. Your digestive system must be in tip top condition for you to have shiny hair and conditioned skin.

Pumpkin seeds are a great source for zinc which in turn limits skin and scalp dryness. Carrots are loaded with vitamin C, although they are predominantly renowned for benefiting the sense of sight. The Vitamin C slows the aging signs, and improves collagen production. Carrot is also rich in vitamin A which limits exaggerated cell development on the outer skin layer.

Almonds are loaded with Vitamin E, which acts as a natural sun shield and antioxidant. Your skin needs a screen which to protect from adverse weather conditions.

39.

Quinoa Alkaline salad recipes

IN ORDER TO LOSE WEIGHT in an effective way, you need to consume more vegetables and high fiber foods that will in turn boost your metabolism. Quality high fiber foods are not in the processed food categories as many would think. Most of the processed foods in the markets labeled as containing high fiber are in fact laden with gluten, sugar and other chemicals. These will thus not assist you in losing weight but will in fact complex your metabolism altogether.

In place of the processed diet, you are advised to consume green leafs, avocado, pepper, black beans, amongst other organic grains and vegetables you might come across. For this particular salad you could throw in jalapeños and tomatoes to add a spicy finish.

South border Quinoa salad

4 servings

Ingredients

- 2 cups of filtered water
- 1 cup Quinoa
- 1 finely diced dell red pepper
- 1 diced full avocado
- 2 tablespoons of chopped cilantro
- 1 15 oz. can of adzuki beans
- 6 tablespoons of virgin olive oil
- 1 tablespoon cumin
- 1 sliced bunch of scallions
- 2 tablespoons of freshly squeezed lemon juice
- Black pepper to taste

- Sea salt to add taste
- ¼ sliced red onion for garnishing (optional)

Directions to follow

Place the quinoa, water a pinch of the sea salt in a medium sauce pan.

Cover and simmer for approximately 15 to 20 minutes.

By the end of this time the water should be fully absorbed.

Remove from stove and set aside

Dressing

In a sizeable bowl combine the extra virgin olive oil, lime juice, and cumin and mix.

Add a pinch of salt and some pepper.

Gently add the quinoa, red bell pepper, adzuki beans, the cilantro and avocado in a fitting bowl and mix well.

Pour the dressing over the mixture of quinoa and toss for coating.

Toss around until all the mixture is well coated by the dressing.

Your healthy alkaline salad is now ready to eat. It can be served warm or cold. Enjoy the meal.

Getting rid of acid

Eating healthy and meaningful yet cost effective diets must be paramount for all. Alkaline salads are not only a sure way of cleansing your body of harmful acid; they assist in shedding weight and energizing your body.

The quinoa salad could also be added with some green leafy vegetables to fully complete the picture of a traditional salad. This however is not mandatory for the salad is well balanced as it is. If the quinoa is prepared beforehand, the salad takes a lesser time to prepare.

The salad is laden with dietary fiber, and minerals such as manganese, phosphorus, copper, magnesium and zinc. Quinoa has antioxidant phytonutrients and two flavonoid, (quercetin and kaempferol) in amounts higher than cranberries. All these phytonutrients are effective anti-inflammatory agents that benefit your body.

Quinoa also contains heart healthy fats in the form of oleic acid and has notable amounts of omega 3. The process of boiling or simmering the quinoa will not have any effects to the fatty acids and you can rest assured that cooking the quinoa will not alter its health benefits to your body.

40.

Health Benefits of the Hemp Plant

HEMP SEEDS AND OILS are a renowned source of Omega 3 fatty acids, and modern usage of hemp includes making of milk, bread, beer, granola bars and cereals. Food products sourced from the hemp seeds will never have similar intoxicant effects as the marijuana although the two are two sides of the same coin. The hemp seeds contain only traces of amounts of THC, the chemical that alters your conscience found in marijuana. The foods on the other side will not have any effects related to marijuana and will not have you testing positive for drug use.

Hemp seeds have been found to contain valuable amounts of Omega 6 to Omega 3 fatty acids amongst other compounds believed to assist in controlling blood pressure. Foods made from hemp seeds are high in fiber, minerals, carbohydrates, proteins; beta-carotene, and Vitamins A, C and E. Beta-carotene are medically proven to reduce premalignant gastric lesions

Studies have shown that hemp seeds also contain sterols, linolenic acids and aliphatic alcohols in its oils which scientists found favorable in controlling coronary heart conditions and cancers. Hemp seeds are easy to prepare as a food and remain highly nutritious when eaten whole.

Recipe for hemp seeds food
Ingredients
- ½ cups of hemp seeds
- A pinch of salt
- 1 teaspoon of extra virgin olive oil
- Red pepper or soy sauce

- Garlic powder or herbs

Directions

Place a dry skillet over medium-high heat.

Pour the hemp seeds into the skillet and stir them till they begin to roast and pop.

At this juncture, turn down the heat and add the olive oil to the seeds.

Stir the olive oil in while seasoning with the salt.

Add the red pepper or soy sauce (as preferred) and keep on stirring.

Add the garlic powder or herbs, and stir.

Eat the food as a healthy snack. It is both nutritious and energy boosting.

You should only prepare as much as you can eat on the go since the seeds are not beneficial kept for long periods of time, they will easily ruin.

Health benefits of the hemp

Hemp grows like a weed but has adverse positive effects in human nutrition for the production of food and other body care products. Scientific records and investigations separate marijuana from the hemp seeds, marijuana contain cannabidiol (CBD) at higher levels than the hemp seeds. This means that marijuana has an added potency of being both a drug and medicine value.

Hemp seeds on the other hand are regarded as nuts in terms of food and nutrition. These seeds contain a savory nutty flavor, making the seeds incredibly versatile for use in baking, cooking, or for adding to salads and smoothies. The seeds are approximately 25 percent protein and also contain other nutrients such as vitamin E, zinc, potassium, calcium, magnesium, phosphorus, iron, and sulfur.

The hemp hearts, as the hemp seeds are popularly referred to as, carry numerous heart healthy compounds, inclusive of some amino acid arginine. Arginine is precursor to nitric acid and has been refuted

by medical studies as to assist in maintaining acceptable blood pressure
levels.

41.

Demystifying nutritional value of Coconut water

COCONUT WATER IS NATURALLY refreshing with a savory nutty flavor and contains electrolytes and easily digested carbohydrates. Many mistake coconut water with the white fluid in fully developed coconuts (coconut milk) or coconut oil. The water in focus here however is the kind which is only obtained from young (green) coconuts. It is a translucent fluid found at the center of the fruit.

The coconut water is low in cholesterol, has natural fats and lesser calories than most refreshments. It is also an optimal hydrant and comes packed with more potassium than four plantains. Coconut water is a sure body hydrant and has medical benefits such as curbing kidney stones, preventing cancer and nurse hangovers.

Coconut water versus sports drinks

Coconut water has less sugar and calories than any soda, sports refreshment and fruit juice. It is recommended for both young and elderly who steer away from sweet beverages, and those who tolerate the nutty flavor. The natural hydrant is laden with potassium and less sodium as compared to any other drink ounce per ounce.

Coconut water is recommended for sports professionals facing long durations of work outs and performances, especially in hot and humid climates. Coconut water can be taken by itself or mixed with ordinary water for effective energy recovery and body rehydration. Coconut water is more efficient in replacing respired body fluids than all other hydrants.

For coconut to effectively replenish your lost body fluids, you have to drink a quantifiable amount altogether. Studies on coconut water have indicated that the fluid is more suitable for athletes since it has minimal to zero secondary effects. It has zero connection to stomach upsets and will not have you nauseating. It is also easier to consume in large quantities for rehydration purposes.

For people engaged in energy demanding prolonged physical commitments, staying well hydrated is most crucial. Coconut water may not go well with many athletes for it has high potassium margins, low on carbohydrates and sodium: which are in high demand by sports professionals' who consistently exercise. It is thus not recommended for those engaged in rigorous and strenuous exercises for durations longer than 3 hours, although it has the same properties as pure water and packaged sports hydrants.

Supplements for sodium levels

There is a need to supplement the intake of sodium and carbohydrates after strenuous exercising, either by consuming a banana or other products like raisins. This is vital since neither the coconut water or sports beverages have adequate sodium and carbohydrates as demanded by your body after much strain and respiration.

Coconut water assists in closing nutritional deficiencies brought on by lack of adequate potassium in the meals you consume. If you lack a balanced diet consistent of fresh vegetables and fruits, you are advised to take coconut water to close the gap left by such inadequacy. Despite reducing sodium content in the body, the coconut water adds enough margins of potassium in the body.

For the average adult who only works out once in a while or exercises less strenuously, it is not paramount to consume the coconut water since ordinary water works out just fine. It is also necessary to note that drinking too much coconut water on the go translates into consuming too many calories at one time.

42.

Liver Cleanse Recipe

A CLEAN LIVER IS ONE of the most basic things you need to live healthier. Well, you can achieve this goal easily with this simple alkaline recipe, and get other health benefits that it comes with too. If you bring on board a few other ingredients, you will be able to supercharge it to get the best out of it. It's always wise that you do this every morning and during the weekends as well. Besides, you need to take a light exercise like jogging before taking your liver cleanse to ensure you flush toxins out of your body and boost the lymph system. Here is the recipe for making this useful liver cleanse juice.

Yield
Servings for 2
Preparation time
10 minutes
Ingredients
2 large grapefruits
4 lemons
300 ml of alkaline or filtered water
2 tablespoons Udo's Choice (you can also use cold pressed flax oil)
1 teaspoon of acidophilus
1-2 cloves of fresh garlic
2 inches of fresh root ginger
A dash of cayenne pepper (optional)
Directions
First, squeeze the grapefruit and lemon juice into a blender

Then add garlic and ginger. Use a garlic press to squeeze them into the juice

Next, add the alkaline water along with the Udo's and acidophilus and blend them for about 30 seconds

Increase the amount of ginger to attain your preferred taste.

Why you need this juice

One thing, the liver cleanse juice is high in liver cleansing contents, which helps the liver to gently but effectively flush and attain self-healing. Besides, it does not pose any risk of side effects, except for the fact that you will experience a bit of garlic-breath for some time after consumption. If you want to suppress this odor, you can always use grapefruit. Another interesting fact about this juice is that it is also useful for a hangover cure, thanks to its rich vitamin C, probiotics, water, omega 3 and ginger contents.

Other health benefits associated with boosting mental function, blood health, hormonal health and immune health. It is also ideal for muscles, skin, eyes, bone, hair and teeth. Besides, it is an antioxidant, and it is efficient for energy and nervous system.

Nutritional Summary

This juice is low in cholesterol or sodium. It is also high in Vitamin A, C, E, K, B6, Folate, and Thiamin. It is also a good source for powerful alkaline salts like Magnesium and Potassium. It is rated as highly Alkaline, with a low Glycemic index of 14, weight loss of 3/5 and optimum health at 3/5.

With the liver being one of the most vital organs in the body, it is important that you make sure it's functioning well. The good news is that since this juice can get you started, achieving this vital step does not have to be a challenge for you. You can start your day with this tasty and healthy drink, which is also quick to prepare, and above all, comes with healthy benefits that any nutritionist will advise you to pursue.

43.

Beneficial Alkaline Herbal Teas

ONE QUESTION THAT PUZZLES many is whether boiled water is alkaline too and the best part is that the answer is yes. Since alkaline water becomes so through ionization or presence of mineral content, its PH boiling does not have any effect on the balance, which makes it even more suitable for making alkaline tea. If you need pH drops, it is advisable that you add them after your tea has boiled and cooled, although this depends on personal preference. Here are the 7 top alkaline drinks for you.

1. Redbush Tea

This tea is high in antioxidants and offers the best alternative to coffee. It tastes quite bitter, which suits for satisfying craving for coffee or black tea, not forgetting that it is packed with nutrients like calcium, zinc, magnesium, and manganese, which are vital alkaline minerals.

2. Yerba Mate Tea

This South American tea comes in handy when you want to detoxify and cleanse. Besides, it offers an energy boost, and it is free from jitters associated with caffeinated drinks like coffee and green tea. This tea contains such vitamins as A, B1, B2, Niacin (B3) B5, B complex, C, and E. It is also rich in minerals like Calcium, Manganese, Iron, Selenium, Potassium, Zinc, Magnesium, and Phosphorous.

3. Peppermint Tea

This type of tea is both tasty and alkaline. It is also great for digestion and refreshing. Besides, it is natural, caffeine-free, and is recommendable for IBS, nausea, heartburn, bad breath and flatulence among other problems.

4. Rosemary Tea

Rosemary is a native of the Mediterranean, and it claims its fair share of recognition among antioxidants. The best part about it is that it is easy to grow, and can be sufficient if well grown. It is high in Vitamin A, B1, B2, Niacin (B3), B6, B12, biotin, and pantothenic acid, Vitamin C, D, E and K. If there is one tea that never disappoints, it has to be this one.

5. Ginger Tea

If you are looking for a solution to indigestion and nausea, then ginger tea is for you. It also comes with benefits like enhancing blood circulation, fighting flu, colds, stress and headaches. This is an ideal drink for the good and bad times.

6. Lavender Tea

Talk about its flavor, relaxing effect and helping you ease into a sound sleep. If you need to reduce stress and anxiety and unwind after a long and tiresome day, then lavender can come to your rescue. Lavender is one of these alkaline teas you cannot afford to miss out on.

7. Rosehip Tea

This may be last, but it is far from being the least. The rosehip is fragrant, tasty and high in nutrient too. It is derived from a wild rose plant fruit, and it is rich in Vitamin C, and several other vitamins, tannins, and minerals. The plant is believed to be an excellent energizer, and high in flavonoids, essential for stronger body capillaries and other benefits. This tea is ideal for flu, colds, headaches and stomachaches, to mention but a few.

These are the seven best alkaline teas that you should try out for better health and tasty drinks anytime. They are not only fragrant and delicious but also offer health benefits that you cannot overlook if you are looking into treating your body well. You have to try them out.

44.

Top 3 Delicious Detox Waters for Body Cleansing and Burn Fat

DETOX IS ONE OF THE best ways to healthy living, and it is possible your physician has already recommended this option. The best part about these drinks is that they are very easy to make and do not require many ingredients, not to mention that you can mix ingredients that match your personal preference. Here are the three best types of detox waters for you.

1. Cucumber, Lemon, and Mint water

How to prepare

Slice the cucumber into pieces

Slice the lemon into rings

Add several mint leaves

Mix all of them in a jar with filtered water

Leave them for about 30 minutes for the ingredients to infuse into the water and enjoy.

Benefits

This water is essential for weight loss since it is a natural appetite suppressant, flushing out toxins and boosting metabolism. It also comes in very handy for healthy skin, dealing with bloating, detoxification of the kidneys and enhancing blood circulation. Additionally, it is also useful for reducing cholesterol, fighting high blood pressure, promoting healthy hair and curbing stomach problems too.

2. Orange and Rose Water

How to prepare

Slice your orange into round rings

Add rose petals

Put them in a jar with filtered water

Leave them for about half an hour and enjoy.

Benefits

This drink is very helpful when it comes to increasing brain function, boosting memory and curbing cravings for sweets. It is also useful for enhancing nutrients, promoting digestion and helping in weight loss as well as promoting healthier skin. Moreover, if you are looking into strengthening your immune system, promoting better digestion and enhancing bowel movement, as well as obtaining sufficient blood pressure regulation and boosting your energy, then this drink is for you.

3. Pineapple and Strawberry Water

How to prepare

Cut your pineapple into thin sections

Cut the strawberry into small fine pieces too

Add them in a jar with filtered water

Sit for about 30 minutes before drinking, for the ingredients to infuse into the water

Take your drink

Benefits

Pineapple and strawberry detox water is very helpful when you are fighting hangover, and when you need to enhance skin nutrients. It is also ideal for keeping you hydrated, and it is high in nutrients that can be very useful in the body too. Besides, this drink is essential for boosting your immune system, anti-inflammatory and better blood circulation too. Pineapple and strawberry detox can also help with anti-ageing, regulating blood sugar and fortifying your colon among other advantages.

You do not have to overthink detox; you can achieve this necessary step without having to spend a fortune. With these three drinks with your diet, or taking them occasionally, you can detox your body without having to face much struggle. Even better, they come with numerous advantages that also count for your overall health, in boosting several body functionalities and increasing nutrient intake too. You can never go wrong with these tasty detox waters.

45.

How to Make Sonoma Chicken Salad

FOR ANYONE WHO LOVES chicken salad, having that nutty, fruity enhanced and honey boosted treat makes this salad special. What counts in this version is the grapes that bring onboard the sweetness, with pecans and celery necessary for crunch, and you can include a little of creamy chive to dress it up. If you want it to taste amazing, you need to look no further than making the chicken with honey, apple cider vinegar and the spices in a crockpot, and the toss it into the dressing the next day. Here are the basics for making this fantastic salad for your family.

Preparation time

35 minutes

Yield

Ingredients

Dressing

1 cup mayonnaise

4 teaspoons apple cider vinegar

5 teaspoons honey

2 teaspoon poppy seeds

¼ teaspoon fine sea salt

Salad

¾ cup of pecan pieces, roasted

2 pounds boneless, it should be skinless chicken breasts

2 cups of red seedless grapes, sliced in half

3 stalks celery, thinly sliced

¼ teaspoon ground pepper

Directions

Mix the mayonnaise, cider vinegar, poppy seeds, pepper, honey and salt in a large bowl. Refrigerate them until they are ready to use. You can do this about 2 days before.

Start by preheating your oven to about 375 degrees F, and then place your chicken breasts in a baking dish, set in one layer and add about ½- cup water. Cover it with foil, and then bake it for about 25 minutes, until well cooked. Now, remove the chicken breasts from the pan and let it cool for about 10 minutes at room temperature. Cover and set in the refrigerator.

Once your chicken is cold enough, slice it into bite-size pieces before transferring into a large bowl. Then add the pecans, celery, grapes and the reserved dressing, while stirring consistently. .

Note

Although it is possible to find a different type of recipe at your local store, it is important to point out that some aspects of flavor, ingredients and allergens can differ from one recipe to the other.

Nutritional value per serving

Serving size about 1 cup

20 g total fat

350 calories (180 from fat)

3g of saturated fat

70 mg cholesterol

420 mg sodium

20 g carbohydrates

2 g dietary fiber

12 g sugar

25 g protein

The best thing about this salad is that as many versions may feature red or green grapes and others have dried cranberries, they are all fantastic. This versatility gives you the choice to swap fruits and nuts, giving you a wider scope for even better and preferable taste. The other upside that comes with this salad is that you can serve it on sandwich bread, scoop it up with crackers, or on a croissant, the Sonoma chicken will always have something for your entire family.

Besides, if you are on a picnic, baby shower or luncheon and you want to throw quite a treat, then this salad can get you on the right track. So go ahead and try your Sonoma chicken salad, whether on monthly basis or more consistently, you will always have a reason to plan for this salad, either regularly or occasionally.

46.

How to Make Gluten-Free Spinach Garlic Tofu Burgers

THIS FOOD IS NOT ALL about what the name suggests, there is more to it, and this is regarding the nutritional value, and health safety as well. There are a lot of things that you can do with spinach and other greens, but when it comes to making the tofu burgers, there is no better way to enjoy this nutritious and healthy veggie. One thing that stands out is that this tofu is gluten- free, which any vegetarian out there would be going for in everything they are consuming. Besides, it also comes with all sorts of benefits, but first, here is a recipe for making this fantastic burger.

Yield

Servings for 2- 4

Ingredients

16 ounces of frozen spinach (should be organic), thawed

¾ cup of gluten free rolled oats

15 ounces firm tofu

A medium onion, chopped

3- 4 big cloves garlic, minced

¼ cup LSA mix

1 tablespoon paprika

Himalayan salt and pepper to taste

1 teaspoon cumin

¼ cup coconut oil

Dash of Bragg Liquid Amino (optional)

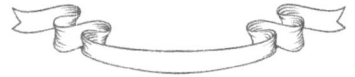

DIRECTIONS

First, crumble the tofu, and then mix all the ingredients in a bowl. Let them sit for several minutes so the oats to absorb a little liquid from the spinach.

Now, add water to the mixture if it is not wet enough for it to combine well, add your Bragg if you wish so.

Create hand-made patties and fry them in coconut oil. If possible, cook for about 6 to 10 minutes on either side and turn them carefully occasionally. Serve your burgers with a big salad.

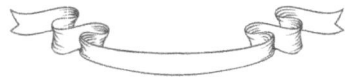

NUTRITIONAL SUMMARY

If there is one sure thing about the spinach garlic, tofu burger is that they are low in both sodium and cholesterol. Besides, they are an excellent source of vitamin C, vitamin A, vitamin K and Folate. They are also known for their rich minerals like Manganese, Magnesium, Calcium, and copper. These burgers are also moderately Alkaline, which makes them an ideal choice for people who are looking for an alkaline meal.

While it is worth noting that the spinach garlic tofu is gluten free, their fresh content cannot be overlooked. Besides, it is also high in important alkaline minerals that you can be sure to boost the pH balance in your body as well. If you like spinach and tofu but just can't figure out the best way to get them going, then you need to look no further, since this is all you need to get on the right track and enjoy them in one bite.

47.

What You Should Know about Herbs and the Alkaline Diet

WHAT YOU SHOULD KNOW about Herbs and the Alkaline Diet

The body PH is an important aspect when it comes to maintaining a healthy living. However, it is essential to understand that herbs play a crucial part in sustaining this balance, especially knowing the benefits of alkaline herbs.

Why are herbs important?

Body balance is optimum at neutral (around 7.0) pH level. With many foods packed with acidic ingredients, it is important to bring onboard an alkaline diet to maintain a healthy balance. This is achieved through the consumption of mostly fruits, nut, veggies, and herbs. Similarly, herbal teas are as important since they are also alkaline-forming. For a diet to be well balanced, it should have about 20 to 40% acid forming foods, and 60 to 80% alkaline forming foods.

What herbs are Alkaline?

1. Turmeric

This is a pungent herb, which has been identified as capable of fighting cancer and inflammation. It can double as food and medicine, thanks to its alkaline properties. It has been confirmed as a feasible treatment for diabetes, ulcers, arthritis, colitis cancer and atherosclerosis. It can be consumed as fresh, or you can get its extract.

2. Cayenne pepper

Almost everyone loves this herb. It is highly alkaline, and ideal for fighting cancer, in weight loss, pain cure, treating arthritis, headaches, and inflammation. You can take it in the form of capsules or consume it fresh.

3. Dandelion greens

These herbs are known to prevent cancer, and are highly alkaline too. They are preferred by many herbalists despite the fact that most people term them as a weed. Their leaves can be added to salads, or used for making herbal tea. The roots can help in treating kidney stones, as they suffice as natural diuretic.

4. Garlic

Talk of a natural antibiotic, anti-viral, antioxidant, or anti-parasitic and you could be well referring to garlic. These traits make garlic chefs and herbalists' a favorite herb, and if you do not like it fresh you can go for tablets or capsules, this herb has everything for everyone.

5. Wheat grass

This herb is added to smoothies, or sometimes consumed as a drink. Wheatgrass is made from young wheat plants, and it offers a good value of alkaline. It is used for the treatment of diseases like a cough, gout, cold, infections, inflammation and cancer among others. Like many other herbs, it can be consumed as an extract or fresh.

Other reliable alkaline herbs include cinnamon, ginger, medical weed, sea vegetables, medical mushrooms and nettles.

Alkaline herbs for teas

Some of the most useful alkaline herbal teas include Rosemary tea, Lavender tea, Rosehip tea, and Peppermint tea among others. Most of these teas are packed with numerous vitamins, important alkaline minerals, and other essential nutrients. They are also useful for treating several diseases and conditions; from simple flu and colds to complicated ones like diabetes and cancer.

With many diseases and imbalances rooted on the condition of the body's environment, it is important to ensure that you keep your balance at its optimum. This can be effective in preventing diseases that thrive in acidic conditions from cancers to colds, and ensuring steady immune system, tissues and well-functioning organs.

48.

Cherry Brown Sugar, with Almonds & Honey

THIS IS A GREAT SUMMER dessert that is easy to whip up and can be combined with several other ingredients as preferred by the consumer. It is a healthy and delicious meal that is a favorite with kids and adults alike. Almonds are not only a great addition to any diet, but they are also considered as effective food products that assist in weight loss.

Almonds are the most nutritious tree nuts as compared to other types of nuts ounce per ounce. The almond nuts are an excellent reservoir for Vitamin E and magnesium, and a remarkable source of dietary fiber and protein.

Cherry has numerous antioxidants and thus is a perfect ingredient for people facing inflammation issues and goiter. As a raw fruit, sweet cherries contain dietary fiber and other vitamins in moderate content.

Cherry brown sugar fool recipe

Ingredients

6 servings

Honey almonds

- 1/3 cups of sliced almonds
- 1 tablespoon honey

Cherry brown sugar fool

- 1 teaspoon of lemon juice
- 1 cup of fresh sweet cherries, pitted
- 1 tablespoon sugar
- ½ tablespoon almond extract

- 1 teaspoon vanilla extract
- 2 tablespoons of light brown sugar
- 2 tablespoons water
- ¾ cups heavy cream

Directions / method

Heat your oven to 400 degrees and place a baking sheet using a baking mat.

Mix the almond nuts in a small bowl with honey.

Spread the honey coated almond nuts on the baking mat and bake them for approximately 7 to 10 minutes. The nuts should by now have turned golden in color.

Transfer the cooked nuts into a different bowl and let them cool.

Once cooled, chop the almond nuts coarsely and set aside.

In a small saucepan, put together the lemon juice, cherries, almond extract, water and sugar.

Cook over medium heating frequently stirring to a degree the cherries commence breaking down. The juices should by now start to boil, cooking should be approximately 5 minutes.

Remove from heat and transfer to a sizeable bowl. Place the small bowl in another bowl of ice water and continue occasional stirring until the food turns cold.

Combine the brown sugar, heavy cream and vanilla and continuously beat until some stiff peaks form. Fold in the 1/3 cup of cherry sauce.

Partially combine the cherry sauce and the stiff peaks from the beat combination. There should be an appearance of beautiful cherry streaks through the fresh cream.

Serve among four dessert dishes while spooning the remainder cherries over top.

Garnish the savory dish with the honey almonds.

Enjoy your delicious dessert.

Nutritional information

Each serving of this astounding summer desert contains 180 calories, (120 of these sourced from fats). The meal is also laden with substantial protein, dietary fibers, saturated fats, sodium, carbohydrates and sugar.

Almonds are considered vegetarian nuts that are recommended for people keen to steering clear of any gluten products. The above recipe caters to about 4 percent of every day nutritional demands by an optimally operating body. Honey assists in the prevention of colds, healing wounds and curb infections. Dark raw honey is also recommended for cases of people keen on limiting sugar consumption in their daily dietary intake.

49.

How to Prepare Avocado and Chickpea Combo

FOR AVOCADO LOVERS, here is another way to get the best out of this amazing fruit. You may have tried all the avocado smoothies out there, but it is possible you have not checked this avocado combo out. The combination of an avocado with chickpeas does not disappoint, especially when you include herbs to spice the whole thing up it adds nutritional value altogether.

What many people find interesting about this food is the fact that it is low in cholesterol and sodium. This enables you to keep the risk of heart diseases and other health problems at bay, while you can still enjoy your delicious combo. If you are yet to try this food, then you need to check it out and take advantage of its rich content for health benefits that you can hardly find in most foods available. Above all, you need to spare only ten minutes of your time, so you also do not have to keep everything else waiting as you make your avocado combo.

Yield

Servings for 2-3

Preparation time

10 minutes

Ingredients

1 can chickpeas, that is drained

A ripe avocado, one is enough

Drizzle of flax oil

Himalayan salt and cracked black pepper

Pinch of cumin

Herbs of your preference, like coriander, basil, parsley (optional)

Directions

Combine the avocado chunks, chickpeas, pepper and salt, cumin and your herbs.

Mash them together, but leave several whole chickpeas

Drizzle the flax oil on top, and the add the paprika before serving

Alternatively, you can put them into your salad wraps or add to your veggies if you want to make your meal more feeling and tastier.

Nutritional Summary

Among the many aspects that make this food exceptional are its low levels of cholesterol. It is also very low in sodium, besides being a reliable source of Vitamin C, Copper, Protein, Calcium, vitamin A, and vitamin K. Further, it is high in alkaline minerals like Magnesium, and Manganese. On alkaline levels, it is rated as moderately alkaline, which is also sufficient for keeping your balance at its optimum.

We all know you can never go wrong with an avocado, especially when it comes to pumping good content into your body. It gets even better when you add the chickpeas into the mix to boost the fiber and protein content into your combo. Besides, since this food is low in cholesterol and sodium, it is an indication that this combo is safe for consumption, even when you want to keep the fear of heart disease out of the question. What's more, when you have such healthy content, you can be sure to stay feeling full for hours. This keeps you out of the cabinets, helping you avoid snacks and compulsive eating habit, especially if you are working on cutting weight. Go ahead and have fun with your delicious avocado and chickpea combo.

50.

Alkaline Avocado Power Shake Recipe

AVOCADO SMOOTHIE ALWAYS comes with something that every nutritionist will recommend for you. This shake not only keeps you full for hours but also has a taste that's smooth and creamy in nature. The best part is this smoothie offers the alkaline portion you need to revitalize your health. If you have not tried this healthy shake, then the time is now.

Yield

Servings for 2

Preparation time

10 minutes

Ingredients

1 cucumber

1 tomato

1 avocado, peeled

1 handful spinach leaves

1 lime, peeled

1 scoop Mega Greens (optional)

10 ml Liquid Chlorophyll (optional)

1 scoop Soy Sprouts (optional)

1 tablespoon Udo's Choice (optional)

Directions

Start by peeling your avocado and lime

Then wash all the ingredients well and slice the cucumber, the avocado, and tomato as well.

Mash your avocado and the stock in a blender and mix them to make a fine paste

Now, add the ingredients with high water content into the blender and mash them into a liquid

Finally, add the spinach, your lime and the supplement that you prefer. Blend them to combine all the ingredients completely

Once everything is ready, serve in a glass.

Nutritional Summary

Avocado shake is low in sodium and cholesterol, and an ideal source of Vitamin B6, vitamin A, vitamin C, vitamin K, Folate, Dietary fiber, and minerals like Potassium and Manganese. It is also highly alkaline and provides about 97% of proteins that you need. On weight loss and maximum health ratings, it has 4/5 and 5/5 respectively. It is also an antioxidant, energizing, good for mental function, muscles, and bones. Besides, it is sufficient for hormonal health, skin, teeth, hair, eyes, blood health and nervous system as well.

The importance of adding the Mega Greens and the liquid Chlorophyll is that they help the drink become even more powerful as a nutritional smoothie.

If you are looking for a great way to start your day, then this shake is for you. Besides keeping you full for hours, you will get sufficient nutritional content with long lasting benefits. With today's diet almost comprising of acidic content, an alkaline smoothie can come in handy to ensuring you maintain the necessary PH balance you need to stay healthy, and most importantly, ensure your immune system is at its best.

Moreover, what most people find interesting about the alkaline avocado shake is that you are at liberty to modify the ingredients as you wish and still get a unique content and taste. What's more, you do not have to spend the whole day making this morning drink, it only takes ten minutes of your time, and you have an entire glass to start your day.

Many people see consuming veggies in the morning as awkward, but this is just as normal if you can get yourself a glass of this smoothie, with a splash of spinach, tomatoes and other greens in the mixture, you can never go wrong with this drink if you want to boost your vegetable intake. The avocado alkaline smoothie never disappoints, you can try it for yourself.

"Let food be thy medicine and medicine be thy food."

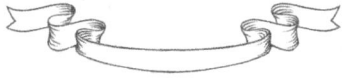

— HIPPOCRATES

51.

What You Should Know about Tamarind and its Benefits

TAMARIND IS A HARDWOOD tree that is native of Africa but still thrives in other areas like Pakistan, India and other countries. This tree's products are bean-like pods with seeds in a fibrous pulp that is sweet sour in taste. These fruits offer different nutrients and health benefits that any physician would recommend for you.

Forms of Tamarind

Tamarind comes in different forms like sweetened syrup and candy, but as a pure fruit, they are also available in various forms too.

Pressed block, which involves removal of the shell and seeds, and compressing the pulp into a block. These are almost like raw tamarind.

Raw pods; as the most natural form of the fruit. While still intact, they can be opened to retrieve the pulp.

Concentrate, which is a boiled pulp. This can be combined with preservatives for longevity.

Uses of tamarind

Tamarind is used in various ways, from health to cooking to household use, thanks to its versatility.

Cooking

This is usually prominent in the South and Southeast Asia, Caribbean, Mexico and the Middle East, since the leaves and seeds of the tree are edible as well. This use comprises marinades, sauces, drinks, desserts and chutneys among others.

Medicine

In medicine, tamarind plays an important role such as past use to treat diarrhea, fever, constipation and peptic ulcers, while the leaves and bark helped with fast wound healing. In the modern world, the plant is under study for possible medicinal uses, with its potent anti-inflammatory and antioxidant properties among other factors. It is also capable of protecting against such diseases as cancer, diabetes and heart diseases.

Domestic use

Due to its tartaric acid property that helps in removing tarnish on copper and bronze, this plant has been used as a metal polish.

Nutritional content

This plant is rich in several types of nutrients, with vitamins B1 (thiamin), vitamin B2 (riboflavin), vitamin and B3 (niacin). It is also high in minerals like Potassium, Magnesium, Phosphorous, Iron, and Calcium. Others like vitamin C, K, B6, B5, and folate are also found in this plant, although in trace amounts, as well as minerals copper, and selenium.

Benefits of Tamarind

Antioxidants

This fruit also contains polyphenols as flavonoids that can help in reducing cholesterol. According to a study, Tamarind fruit extract can lower bad cholesterol LDL and triglycerides. It can also assist in reducing oxidative damage to LDL cholesterol, which contributes to heart diseases.

Antifungal, antiviral and antibiotic effects

This fruit further contains natural compounds that exhibit antimicrobial effects. Studies have also shown that this plant could have antifungal, antibacterial and antiviral activity. Besides, it has been in use as a traditional medicine to treat malaria and other diseases.

Tamarind is one of the plants out there that you may not recognize, but the benefits that can be far reaching. However, this fruit may contain unsafe levels of lead, which may pose a danger to children and expectant women, and can damage the kidney and nervous system too. Therefore, as many benefits as this plant has, it is wise noting that it also comes with its fair share of shortcomings. Thus it should be handled cautiously.

52.

Oregano; Benefits and Side Effects

OREGANO IS ONE OF THE herbs renowned for their culinary and medicinal benefits, with its fair share of health benefits. This herb grows only 50 cm tall, with purple leaves at about 2 to 3 cm long. The herb has a particular smell, thanks to thymol, limonene ocimene, caryophyllene, and carvacrol and pinene chemicals. This herb goes beyond being a useful flavor herb, to containing antioxidants and antibacterial properties. Here are some of the benefits of oregano and its shortcomings too.

Antibacterial and anti-inflammatory

This herb contains antimicrobial tendencies, with some researchers finding out that Origanum vulgare oils are effective against up to 41 food pathogens. The antimicrobial potency of the herb further comes from its carvacol chemical. Besides, a study has also shown that this herb has an active ingredient, beta-caryophyllin, which can be used against osteoporosis, arteriosclerosis and other disorders. According to a study by British and Indian researchers, Himalayan oregano contains strong antibacterial properties capable of killing superbug MRSA.

Cancer protection

A survey carried out in the United Arabs Emirates has shown that oregano has anticancer activity, influenced by encouraging cell cycle arrest, as well as apoptosis, which is effective in cases of breast cancer. The herb also exhibits tendencies to slow down or prevent progression of the disease. Therefore, researchers have concluded that oregano can suffice as a therapeutic candidate for moderating such cancerous cases.

High in essential Vitamin K

Besides containing antioxidants and other benefits, oregano is also an excellent source of vitamin K, which is important in promoting bone growth, maintaining bone density and boosting production of blood clotting proteins as well.

Other benefits

The list of advantages that goes with oregano is an amazing benefit for health, from being able to counter diseases and conditions like bronchitis, cold, muscle pain, toothache, bloating, intestinal parasites, fatigue, menstrual cramps allergies, and heart conditions. Others include a cure for headaches, earache, dandruff, acne, and repelling insects, to mention just a few.

Side effects

Among the side effects of the use of oregano are causing stomach upsets in some when eaten. For allergic people who do not fare well with plants belonging to the Lamiaceae family like mint, sage, basil and others may also be prone to the allergic reaction if upon eating this herb.

There goes your oregano, a mild herb with high power to heal notorious diseases and other complicated conditions. This herb also doubles as a great food spice, which means it is readily available and easy to include into your diet. If you have only been using it to increase the pleasant flavor and taste of your foods, now you know that there is more to look for in this herb than just spicing your diet. However, it is worth noting that oregano may not be appropriate for everyone, which calls for caution. If you are not sure, whether this herb can be useful for you, consulting with your physician or nutritionist could help know where to start.

53.

Top Eleven Benefits of Chia Seeds

CHIA SEEDS ARE DERIVED from Salvia Hispanica, a South American plant related to mint. These seeds have been in use for a long time, and their content and nutritional value has been outstanding. Lately, they have graduated into a modern super food. These seeds are high in nutrients like fiber, proteins, fat, and such minerals as Manganese, Calcium, Magnesium, and Phosphorous. Further, they contain traces of Zinc, Vitamin B, B3, and B2. What's more interesting is the fact that these seeds are low in calories, with only 137 in one ounce, while they also pack a gram of digestible carbohydrates.

1. Most of their carbohydrates are fiber

In one ounce of chia seeds, you get 12 grams of carbs. The best part is that 11 of the total grams are fiber that the body does not digest. However, this does not raise blood sugar, thus does not necessitate disposition of insulin, which cancels it out as carbohydrate. This fiber absorbs a lot of water and keeps you feeling full for long, which can help if you are working on reducing weight.

2. Potent with antioxidants

These seeds are also known for their high levels of antioxidants, which prevent the sensitive fats in the seeds from becoming rancid. Besides, these antioxidants are useful for health, although they can lead to free radicals that damage cells and result in aging and dangerous diseases.

3. High quality protein

Chia seeds have about 14% protein on their weight, which surpass the level in many plants. They also have significant levels of amino acids, which makes their protein content viable for the human body.

4. Help in weight loss

The high protein and fiber content in chia seeds is the secret that can be unleashed to achieving effective weight loss. Protein is effective in suppressing appetite and thoughts about food, while fiber absorbs water and keeps you feeling satisfied for long.

5. They are rich in bone nutrients

Several nutrients in chia seeds like calcium, magnesium, phosphorous and protein are crucial for bone health. The good news is that these seeds contain higher levels of calcium, even than most dairy products; hence they can be a good replacement supplement or alternative calcium source.

6. They improve blood markers and reduce risk of diseases

Chia seeds are rich in protein, fiber, and omega-3, which is essential for metabolism. When combined in a diet with oats, nopal, and soy protein, chia seeds have shown an impressive effect in lowering LDL cholesterol and triglycerides, thus increasing HDL cholesterol and reducing inflammation as a result. All these have proved effective for these seeds to reduce the risk of heart diseases and other diseases.

7. Abundant Omega -3 fatty acids

These seeds are also high in omega-3, even higher than sea fish like salmon. The only downside is that their omega-3 is mostly ALA that is not that much beneficial to the body. This is because ALA has to be converted into active forms like EPA and DHA for it to take effect in the body, and yet the body is incapable of making the conversion. These acids can be found in other sources like fish instead.

8. Can help fight Type 2 Diabetes

Studies have proven that chia seeds are effective against this type of diabetes, thanks to their improvements on some of the most significant health markers. They have been confirmed to lower blood pressure and inflammation as well.

9. They can help in exercise

Just like sports drinks are effective in a workout, chia seeds are believed to be an ideal option too. This is according to a recent study, in which these seeds were tested against Gatorade, and proved efficient in offering athletes enough carb load to keep going, with an increased nutrient boost and lowered sugar intake.

10. Chia seeds are easy to include into your diet

This may not be necessarily a health benefit, but it is undisputable anyway. These seeds tend to get along with different types of foods, and they can be ground too for increased versatility.

These are the chia seeds and their benefits. Maybe you have never figured out they can be essential, but now you know what they are capable of, if you are looking into boosting your health with diet, then this could be the solution for you.

54.

Kale Chips for Energy

MAKING KALE CHIPS MAY be a bit tricky but once you strike a balance you can prepare crispy but chewy kales without having burnt edges. If you can bake them quite well, you can make the best chips ever.

1. Removing the stems and tearing the leaves

You may have your own style of doing this, but when you have kales to pluck from their stems, it does not have to be that complicated. All you need is to hold the leaf on one hand and the stem on the other, and pull them apart, sliding the leaf off the stern.

2. Wash and dry the leaves

Water in the leaves can steam your kale chips while baking, and make them soggy. To avoid this, make sure you dry your leaves well before applying the oil. This can be done on a salad spinner, with keeping an eye on the loading to ensure the leaves dry properly.

3. Bring some oil onboard

Use coconut oil or extra virgin oil to bake. Using about ½ tablespoon of the oil on each baking sheet can be handy, especially in helping the spices stick to the leaves. Apply just enough to cover the nooks and crannies, but do not drench them.

4. Apple to layer after the other

If you do not want your kale chips to become soggy and unevenly baked, avoid dumping all of them onto the baking sheet. Just take your time and spread a layer after another, and remember to rotate the sheet halfway through your baking. If you have time on your side, you can flip the chips over, otherwise, only proceed one way.

5. Maintain minimum heat

Do you want your kale chips to be impressive? Ensure to bake them at low temperatures, 300 F for ten minutes and rotating your pan and cooking for about fifteen more minutes does the trick quite well. Although this may take a while longer than higher heat, it is always important to get the best results. Otherwise, you will end up with scorched kale and not the crispy taste you wanted.

6. Leave them on the baking sheet to cool for a few minutes

To get crispier chips, leave them for about 3 minutes once you get them from the oven. Although the wait may be a hard one, being patient gives them some time to firm up as they cool.

55.

Top Four Rosemary Teas, and Tips on making them

ROSEMARY IS AN HERB among the mint family that is high in fiber, iron, antioxidants carsonol and carsonic acid. It also contains rosmarinic acid, caffeic acid, betulinuc acid and ursolic acid, to mention a few. These natural acids are useful for memory and brain support. Besides, this herb is mood enhancing, antibacterial, anti-inflammatory and stimulating. The herb just comes with almost all types of advantages. Well, here are the top 4 types of rosemary tea that you can use for these benefits and more.

1. Rosemary tea with honey

Ingredients

1 to 2 springs fresh rosemary (or about 1.5-teaspoon dry rosemary)

3-teaspoon honey

2 cups boiling water or 500 ml cold tap water

Directions

You can brew your tea as normal, by boiling the rosemary pieces in water for 8 minutes. You can give it a longer time, and then add some honey. Alternatively, you can simmer the herb in a saucepan to get a stronger taste. This starts by boiling it along with water and honey, and then reducing the heat and leaving it to cook for about 5 minutes. You may press your rosemary against the pan to extract its juices.

2. Rosemary tea with milk

Ingredients

1-cup milk

1 sprig fresh rosemary/ 1 teaspoon dry rosemary

1-teaspoon honey

Directions

Quarter the rosemary, then put three pieces into a saucepan with milk and heat to boil. Reduce the heat and let simmer for about five minutes, stirring consistently to avoid developing a smoky taste. Remove from heat, and discard the rosemary you used to boil, and then put the remaining quarter on top of your tea. You can include honey if you want to make an energizing drink.

3. Rosemary, lemon peels, and ginger

Ingredients

1 bunch of rosemary

1 inch sliced ginger

½ lemon peels

2 cups water

2-teaspoon honey

Directions

Boil all the ingredients in water for eight minutes. You can also cook them in a saucepan and simmer for 6 minutes in case you want a stronger taste. Strain your tea and add honey to taste, and enjoy.

This tea is rich in antioxidants and minerals and can help ease flu symptoms, cold, bronchitis and clearing phlegm.

4. Mediterranean rosemary tea, with sage, thyme, cinnamon and honey

Ingredients

2 cups of water

2 large sprigs rosemary, fresh

2 teaspoon of sage

1-teaspoon thyme

1 cinnamon bark/ ½-teaspoon ground cinnamon

2-teaspoon honey

Directions

In a saucepan, bring water to boil and add all the ingredients. Let simmer for 8 minutes over low heat to be ready.

These ingredients are high in antioxidants and minerals, and can help with flu, cold and keeping warm.

These rosemary teas are not only high in nutrients, minerals, and antioxidants; they are as well easy to make from natural and available herbs. They also take a short time to prepare, which means they can be a great way to start your day, especially if you want to stay energized throughout the day. Make your favorite rosemary tea and enjoy the tasty and healthy benefits that come with this tea, you will love it. Rosemary always has a reason to impress.

56.

How to Prepare Alkaline Tom Yum Soup

A FLAVORFUL, TASTY and healthy soup is not as simple to make, as it may be fun to enjoy. However, if well made, you can get a combination of ingredients that are not only pleasing to the eye but also appealing to your sense of smell and taste as well, not to mention that it comes with as many benefits too. The alkaline Tom Yum soup is one of the best choices you can make, and the healthiest you can put on your table. This soup comes with numerous benefits, various ingredients, and above all, you can find it quite easy to prepare. If you are looking into trying it, this recipe can be useful.

Yield

Servings for 2

Preparation time

25 minutes give or take

Ingredients

1 stick lemongrass

1 or 2 red chili

½ brown onion, sliced into large chunks

2 small Galangal strips

2 small strips of fresh ginger

2 kefir lime leaves

2 cloves garlic

2 quartered tomatoes

Coriander, a handful

Soy sauce, or Bragg Liquid Amino's (you can use Bragg, as it is more alkaline)

600 ml vegetable stock from vegetable Bouillon/ yeast-free stock cubes

Tofu, to your preferred level

Directions

Start by preparing all the flavors. Then, chop several thin ginger and galangal strips, cut the chili stem off, and cut it with the knife, no need to chop. Next, cut your 1.5-inch pieces of the lemongrass and bash it too. Similarly, smash your garlic, and rip off the lime leaves into two halves.

Next, place your spicy pieces into a pot along with the other ingredients and your onions. Bring them to a boil before adding the tofu. Let cook for about two minutes before adding your tomatoes, and then leave them for one more minute before putting in the coriander and the bean sprouts (these sprouts are optional). After adding these, remove from the oven and serve.

Your alkaline Tom soup will be hot, and delicious, but if you want to make it even tastier but less in alkali content, you can splash in some brown sugar, a pinch can do. Then season it with pepper and salt.

Nutritional summary per serving

This food is low in cholesterol, and as well low in sodium. It offers a significant supply of Protein, Vitamin A, vitamin K, vitamin C, Vitamin B6, and Folate. It is also high in minerals like Potassium, Magnesium, Iron, Phosphorous, Copper, Manganese and Calcium.

The taste may be great, but it is just the tip of the iceberg when you come to think of the health benefits in this soup. Besides, you are at liberty to fine tune your ingredients and seasoning to make your soup a required taste, as you prefer, which makes it exceptionally fast to prepare, making it simple and versatile to cover for diverse preferences.

57.

How to make Ginger and Leafy Greens Stir-Fry

IF YOU ARE A LOVER of stir-fry and need more of nutritional content, here is something for you. This stir-fry is a great way to enjoy several leafy greens, from cavalo nero, spinach, green cabbage, to chard, which come with significant nutrients. Besides, they are also packed with dietary fiber, vitamin C, vitamin K, Iron, Calcium, folic acid and many other beneficial nutrients that can make the difference in your health. If you think of making this amazing fry, then this recipe can be useful.

Yield

Servings for 2

Ingredients

½ squash, scoop the seeds out, cut it into 1 cm pieces (peel the skin in case of the squash with a thick skin)

1 finely sliced onion

1-2 cm peeled and chopped ginger piece

¼ cabbage (can be Savoy, Green or any other type you fancy)

Several handfuls of leafy greens, chopped (like kale, cavalo nero, spinach or chard. Etc.)

1 green or red chili, finely chopped

2 tablespoons coconut oil (you can also use cold-pressed oils ideal for stir-fries)

½ fresh lemon juice

Celtic sea salt or Himalayan crystal salt

Pepper, freshly ground

Braggs Liquid Aminos, a dash (another alternative to soy sauce)

Some water

Directions

Start by heating your coconut oil in a large pan or frying pan. Over low heat, cook the onions gently for a couple of minutes. Add your ginger, garlic, and the chili, and continue cooking for about a moment, keeping an eye to ensure the ginger is not burnt since it can get bitter.

Next, add your squash along with a pinch of salt. Fry them gently, cooking the squash to become tender.

Now, toss the leafy greens in and splash in a little lemon juice. Then add a dash of Braggs Liquid Aminos before seasoning with pepper to your preferred taste. The greens take about one to two minutes to cook to ensure you retain their freshness, flavor and the nutrients too. Enjoy your healthy ginger and leafy green stir-fry.

This food is significantly alkalizing, thanks to the squash, which is also a good source of several vitamins. The squash is high in Vitamin A, vitamin C, vitamin K, and vitamin E. Besides, it is rich in alkalizing minerals like Magnesium, Iron, Potassium, and antioxidants.

The ginger and leafy greens stir-fry is a great way of pumping nutrients and minerals into your diet, quickly and conveniently. Besides, since the ingredients and spices here are all natural, you can be sure to get these benefits without the fear of posing a grave danger to your health. This fry-stir is thus an ideal source of delicious and flavorful way of enjoying your greens and squash.

It also offers an appropriate way of keeping the non-organic foods that could be detrimental to your health at bay. If you love squash and veggies, then this stir fry is for you. What's even more attractive, its preparation is pretty easy and takes only a few minutes of your time, so you do not have to worry about sacrificing your precious time with the family to be in the kitchen. Go ahead and try it out.

58.

How to make Avocado Margaritas

IF YOU LOVE HAVING your bread or crackers along with something else, then you need to try this natural spread. It is an ideal combination of ingredients from natural veggies and fruits, as well as spices, which assures the best regarding health and taste. This spread is also alkaline, above all the other benefits that it comes with, that surpass many other main meals.

Yield

Servings for 2

Preparation time

1o minutes

Ingredients

2 cups of peas (either fresh or frozen, can do well with freezing)

1 cup broad beans (fresh or frozen, padded)

1/3 avocado

1/3 cup olive oil or flax oil

1 clove garlic

Celtic sea salt or Himalayan salt to taste (about ½ teaspoon can do)

Fresh mint, a handful

Coriander, 3 springs

1 lemon, juiced (and a rind of half of the lemon)

Directions

Start by washing the peas together with the broad beans. Then boil them for about two minutes

Next, put your boiled beans into a coriander, and then wash with cold water

Blend your beans in a food processor or blender, along with the coriander, avocado, garlic, oil, mint, salt and your rind.

Add some lemon juice to the mixture

Nutritional summary per serving

This food is very low in cholesterol and sodium as well. However, it is a great source of Vitamin A and vitamin K, as well as Dietary Fiber.

And there goes your soft, tasty and healthy spread. It will leave you feeling full, so you will not have to hit the cabinets anytime soon for more, and that could help if you are keeping your weight under check.

If there is one thing that stands out about this spread is that it features several contents that are high in nutritional value, and yet it does not pose a risk for heart diseases, thanks to the low cholesterol and sodium. Besides, with the dietary fiber and all those other health benefits, you can be sure to be on the healthy side with this spread. And remember, you can as use it as a dip with some fresh veggies too.

59.

How to make an Alkalizing Catalan Stew

WHEN IT COMES TO MAKING stew, you need to ensure that the stew you bring to the table is not only tasty and flavorful but also healthy. This is where the alkalizing Catalan stew comes in, to give you more than just the taste, but also some additional benefits that count for overall good health. One thing that makes this stew one of a kind is the fact that it features several veggies and fish among other ingredients, bringing you the best combination proteins and other constituents of safe and healthy contents.

It is understood that its alkalizing effect is outstanding, which comes in handy for helping your body maintain the necessary PH balance. It is also worth noting that Alkaline-rich foods are not only good for your body PH, but also contribute to helping the liver flush and heal itself seamlessly, and other benefits to the kidney as well. Here is the recipe for making the alkalizing Catalan stew, which can be an excellent way to offer a special treat to your family occasionally.

Yield

Servings for 4

Ingredients

6 tablespoons olive oil

1 chopped large Spanish onion

2 chopped fennel bulbs

1 finely chopped red chili

1 teaspoon ground fennel seeds

2 crushed cloves new season garlic

½ teaspoon of sweet paprika powder

1 tablespoon of fresh thyme leaves

1-teaspoon saffron strands

3 bay leaves, fresh

1 tin of plum tomatoes

250 ml/ 3½ fl. oz. water or fish stock

650 g 1 lb. 7 oz. filleted, Tofu or firm white fish (Pollock, cod, bream, monkfish)

100g/ 3 ½ oz. ground toasted almonds

1 lemon, chopped into wedges

Spring Greens and Quinoa

Directions

In a large pan, heat the water, and steam the onions, chili, the ground fennel seeds, fennel, and garlic, for several minutes.

Next, add your paprika, along with the saffron, bay leaves, thyme, and tomatoes. Cook until they become a thick sauce.

Now, add your fish stock or the water and let it heat until simmer.

Add your tofu or the fish pieces into the sauce, and then put the almonds, stirring consistently.

Leave them in the heat for about one or two minutes before serving with the quinoa, seasonal greens, and your lemon wedges.

Nutritional summary per serving

One sure thing about this food is that it is low in sodium, and even very low in cholesterol. It is also a good source of Calcium, Vitamin C, and Manganese.

Since this stew is low in sodium and cholesterol alike, it is an assurance that it is not only efficient for delicious taste but us also a safe way to enjoy your meal without fearing for your health. Since these two can have far reaching effects on your heart and lead to other health complications, it is always a great way of ensuring that you get the potent contents in into your body safely. Besides, since it features several veggies in the mix, it is a sure thing that there is a lot that you can benefit from, not to mention that it is easy to prepare, so you can make it almost any time, even when time is not on your side.

60.

Almost Alkaline Fajitas Recipe

ALKALIZING RECIPES are diverse, and most of them feature different ingredients. However, the results are quite the same, with all of them offering an alkalizing effect essential for your overall health, besides helping with your pH balance, and purification of the liver and the kidneys.

The fajitas could be all you need to make the difference in your diet list, coming with several vegetables that are potent with nutritional values you can hardly find anywhere else. Additionally, they also feature fruits like avocado, bringing on board a combination of dietary sources, taste, and several spices for flavor sum everything up.

Yield

Servings for 2

Preparation time

20 minutes

Ingredients

Wheat Tortillas sprouts (or you can get any healthy wraps available)

1 avocado

1 tomato

Spinach, a handful

1 carrot, grated

1 red onion

1 tablespoon coriander, fresh

Olive oil

1 can of kidney beans

Lettuce leaves, a handful

Pine nuts, a handful

Directions

Start by making salsa for the wraps. Finely chop the tomato and red onion, and then mix them with olive oil. Leave it to infuse.

In the meantime, steam the broccoli lightly until soft enough, then mash it up, and add it to the wrap along with the avocado and salsa. Now, add your spinach, together with the pine nuts, lettuce leaves, and the grated carrot. If you are using the kidney beans, warm them a bit and mash them a little before adding. Besides, you can add some jalapenos into the mixture as well.

There goes your almost alkaline recipe. Call it tasty, realistic, and flavor- filled treat for your family, you can never go wrong with this recipe. What I find most interesting about it is that it is not only delicious and filling, but is also quite easy to prepare, and takes only several minutes and you are done.

Most important noting is the fact that this recipe also gives you the liberty to switch ingredients to fit your excellent taste or make use of what you can find. This is an added advantage for those who are out of reach for some of the ingredients or those who just love experimenting in the kitchen.

References

"Man know thyself"

MARIA ANGELES FERNÁNDEZ-Arche et al "Hemp (Cannabis sativa L.) Seed Oil: Analytical and Phytochemical Characterization of the Unsaponifiable Fraction," Journal of Agricultural and Food Chemistry, DOI: 10.1021/jf404278q

41. Vartanian LR, Schwartz MB, Brownell KD. Effects of soft drink consumption on nutrition and health: a systematic review and meta-analysis. Am J Public Health. 2007;97:667-75.

46. Malik VS, Popkin BM, Bray GA, Despres JP, Willett WC, Hu FB. Sugar-sweetened beverages and risk of metabolic syndrome and type 2 diabetes: a meta-analysis. Diabetes Care. 2010;33:2477-83.

47. de Koning L, Malik VS, Kellogg MD, Rimm EB, Willett WC, Hu FB. Sweetened beverage consumption, incident coronary heart disease, and biomarkers of risk in men. Circulation. 2012;125:1735-41, S1.

48. Fung TT, Malik V, Rexrode KM, Manson JE, Willett WC, Hu FB. Sweetened beverage consumption and risk of coronary heart disease in women. Am J Clin Nutr. 2009;89:1037-42.

49. Choi HK, Willett W, Curhan G. Fructose-rich beverages and risk of gout in women. JAMA. 2010;304:2270-8.

50. Choi HK, Curhan G. Soft drinks, fructose consumption, and the risk of gout in men: prospective cohort study. BMJ. 2008;336:309-12.

51. Hu FB. Resolved: there is sufficient scientific evidence that decreasing sugar-sweetened beverage consumption will reduce the prevalence of obesity and obesity-related diseases. Obes Rev. 2013;14:606-19.

52. Schulze MB, Manson JE, Ludwig DS, et al. Sugar-sweetened beverages, weight gain, and incidence of type 2 diabetes in young and middle-aged women. JAMA. 2004;292:927-34.

53. Palmer JR, Boggs DA, Krishnan S, Hu FB, Singer M, Rosenberg L. Sugar-sweetened beverages and incidence of type 2 diabetes mellitus in African American women. Arch Intern Med. 2008;168:1487-92.

54. Malik VS, Schulze MB, Hu FB. Intake of sugar-sweetened beverages and weight gain: a systematic review. Am J Clin Nutr. 2006;84:274-88.

54. http://www.marshfieldclinic.org

55. http://www.oklahomagardening.okstate.edu/recipes

56. http://oklahomagardening.okstate.edu

57. http://sditlapj.blogspot.com/2012/02/alkaline-recipies.html

58. http://food-nutrition.knoji.com

59.www.wholefoodsmarket.com

60. http://incrediblerecipe.com

61. http://liveenergized.com

62. http://pdfpedia.com/

63. Hulkower, Raphael (2010). "The History of the Hippocratic Oath: Outdated, Inauthentic, and Yet Still Relevant". The Einstein Journal of Biology and Medicine. 25/26: 41–44.

64. "Edwin Smith Papyrus". Turning the Pages Online. U.S. National Library of Medicine Communications Engineering Branch. February 25, 2015.

65. The Papyrus Ebers: The Greatest Egyptian Medical Document. Translated by Ebbell, Bendix. Copenhagen: Levin & Munksgaard. 1937. LCCN 37020036

66. http://www.medicalnewstoday.com/

67. Healing tea. (Reader Remedy)(Brief article
AUTHOR: Boivin, Marie-Claude
BODY:

To fight bacteria, colds, and flu, as well as asthma and allergy symptoms, try this homemade tea. Brew together in one cup of water: 1 clove, 1/2 teaspoon of sage, 1/2 teaspoon of thyme, 1 cinnamon stick, 1/4 teaspoon of cayenne pepper, the juice of half a lemon, and 1 teaspoon of honey.

Marie-Claude Boivin Sherbrooke, Quebec

68. http://www.medicfacility.info/
69. http://www.caringmedical.com/
70. http://www.myhdiet.com/
71. http://nutritiondata.self.com/

WARNING

Remember, always consult with your nutritionist regarding introducing herbs into your diet and specifically discuss any foods that may pose allergy risks for yourself. Some products and claims made about specific products on or through this book have not been evaluated by the United States Food and Drug Administration and are not approved to diagnose, treat, cure or prevent disease. The information provided in this book is for informational purposes only and is not intended as a substitute for advice from your physician or other health care professional or any information contained on or in any product label or packaging. You should not use the information in this book for diagnosis or treatment of any health problem or for prescription of any medication or other treatment. You should consult with a healthcare professional before starting any diet, exercise or supplementation program, before taking any medication, or if you have or suspect you might have a health problem. Not responsible for typographical errors or misprints.

www.ingramcontent.com/pod-product-compliance
Lightning Source LLC
Chambersburg PA
CBHW060517290526
45791CB00001B/420